Introduction

This workbook is designed to help practical therapists understand the many different reflected points and pathways that exist all over the body. It is considered that there are as many as 14 reflected areas that may be used for analysis and 10 reflected areas that may be used for treatment.

The areas of analysis are found in the iris, face, tongue, teeth, temple, pulse, hand, skull, ear, foot, abdomen (two types), spine and the meridians. The areas that are used in treatment may be found on the skull, temple, hands, feet, face, abdomen, ears, spine as well as the meridians, plus major and minor chakra points.

Each of the reflected points and pathways that exist on the surface of the body may be likened as 'holographic images' of internal organs, muscles, joints, vertebral levels etc. Whenever part of the body experiences pain, discomfort, trauma or any other form of energy imbalance, the many reflected points or areas (reflexes) become tender. The reflexes are used as guidelines in analysis and treatment and as they become less tender and more relaxed with treatment, the body part too becomes more relaxed. The reflexes represent the microcosm within the macrocosm of the human frame.

For the very first time, many of these reflected energy pathways are shown in a single publication, thus making the task of the physical therapist easier and clearer in the patient's assessment and treatment.

Body and Foot Vertical and Horizontal Zones

This first illustration should be well known to all therapists who use reflexology in any form. Zone therapy is a system of healing that connects the different body sections using invisible dividing lines. The division of ten vertical zones is due to the number of fingers and toes. The thumb and great toe together with the very medial aspect of the body are placed in the most medial zone, whereas the little toe and little finger together with the most lateral aspect of the body are in the outer zone. The other three zones are placed equally between these two. Sensitivity and tension in the reflected area indicates a problem in another part of the zone. In addition to the vertical zones, zone therapy uses horizontal divisions. This has become very useful to reflex therapists in dividing the body into treatable sections on the feet and hands.

Traditionally, the diagram of the vertical body zones is shown with the arms medially rotated so that the thumb approximates the lateral aspect of the thigh.

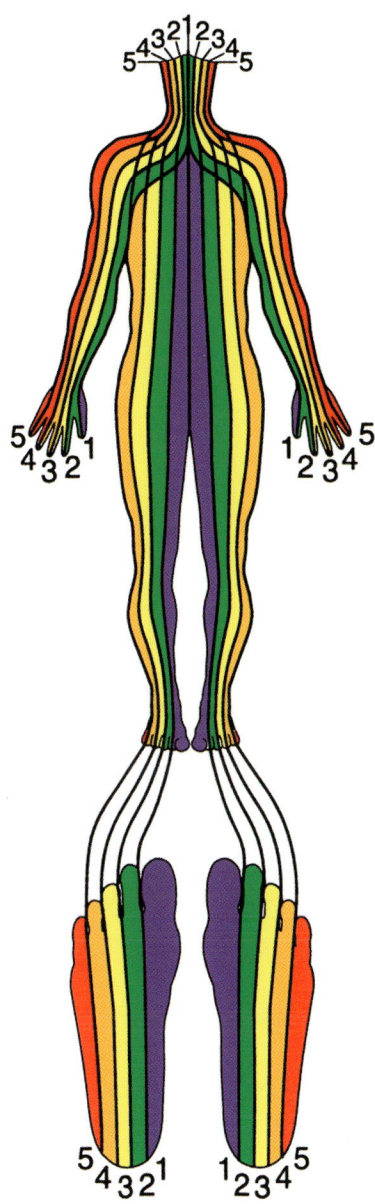

Body and feet zones

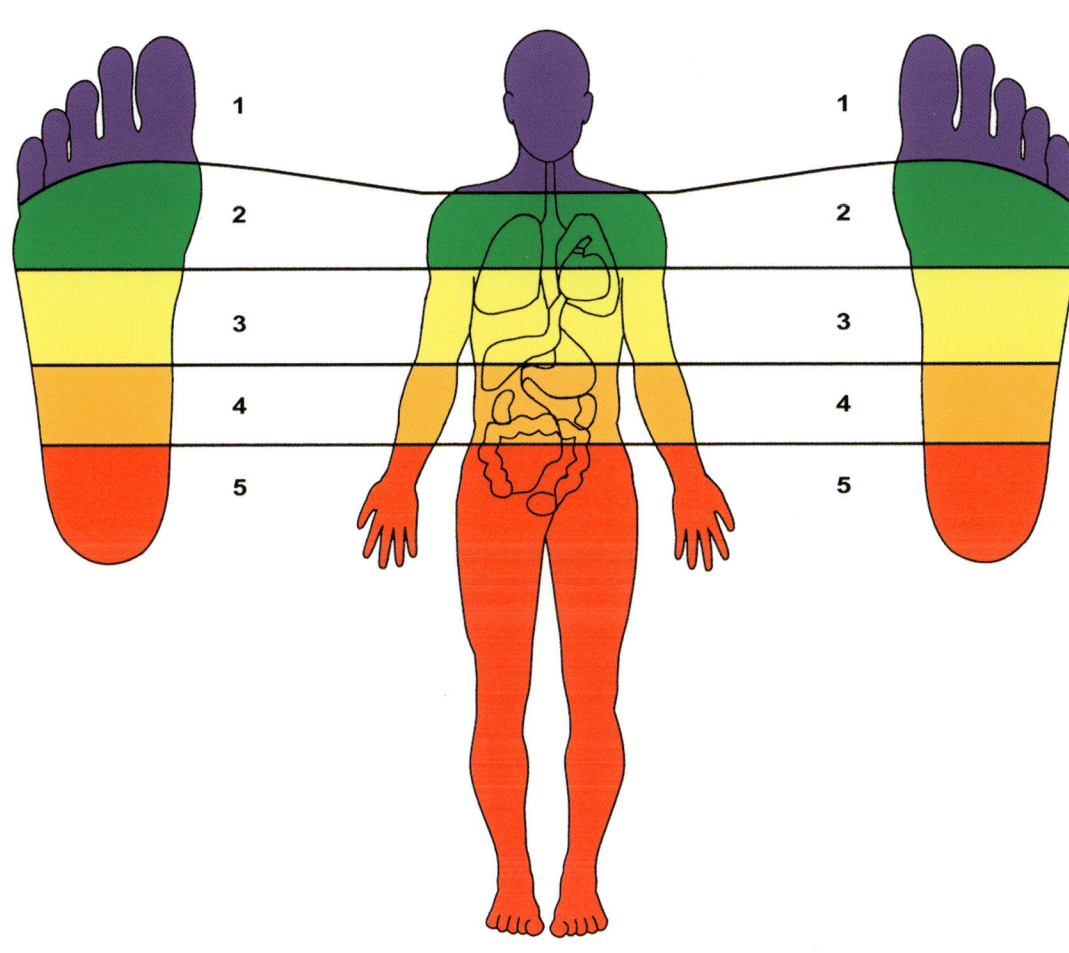

Level of reflexes on the feet

Parallel Areas of the Joints

The principle of parallel joints is based on vertical and horizontal zone therapy. It could also be called parallel zones. In simple terms, if it is impossible to treat part of the body locally due to an open wound or some other contra-indicating disease factor, its parallel reflected area may be treated. The hand is parallel to the foot, the knee is parallel to the elbow, the shoulder is parallel to the hip and the neck is parallel to the pelvis. Taking this one stage further, the thumb is parallel to the great toe, the little finger to the little toe and so on.

As well as treating the parallel area in isolation, an energetic balance may also be attempted between the part of the body that requires treatment and its parallel reflected area. This remains an extremely useful adjunct in reflex therapy. With such large areas to energy balance, it is permissible to place the whole of the hand over each of the joints.

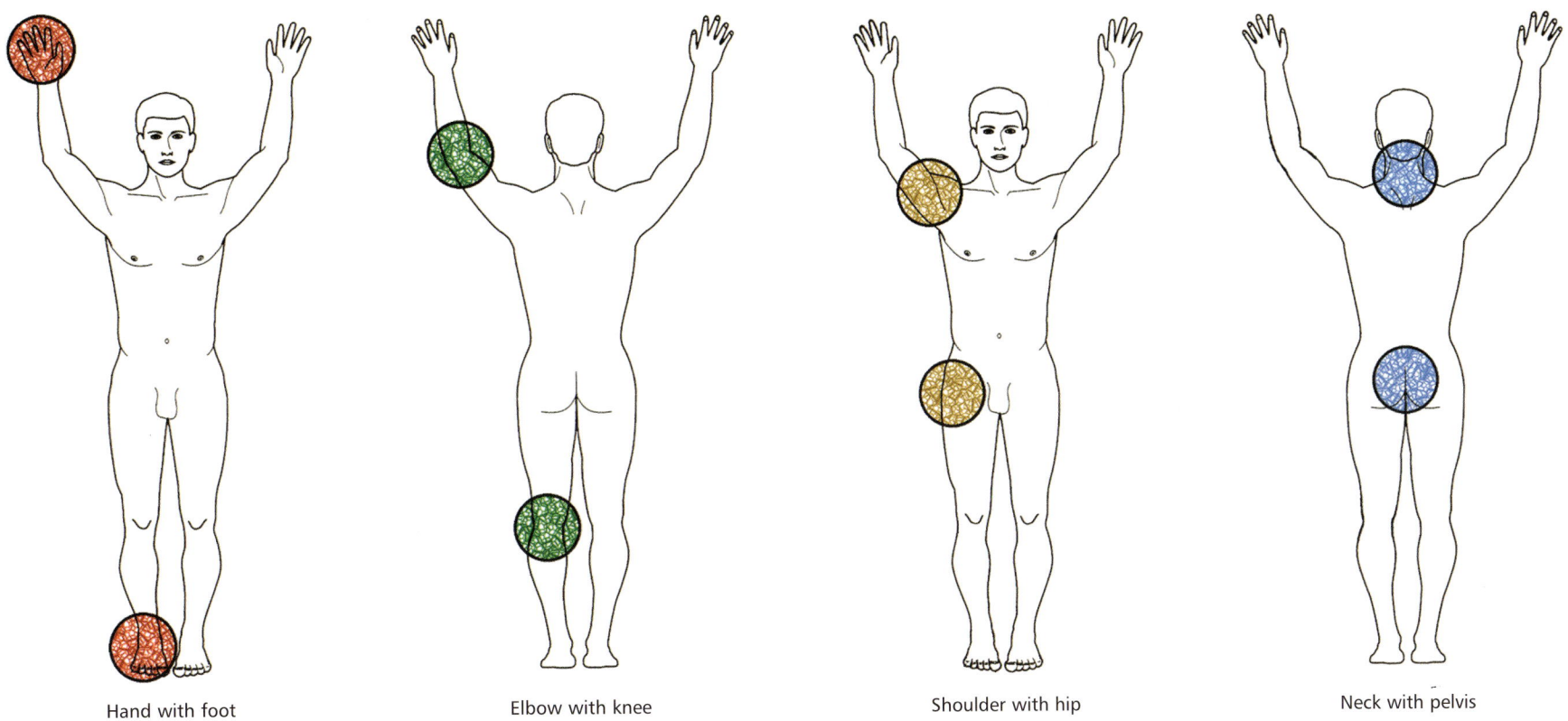

Foot Reflexes

The foot represents the most important area of reflected energy pathways on the body and is the area that is used more than any other. It does, of course, represent a whole treatment paradigm in Foot Reflexology. It has its roots in Traditional Chinese Medicine (TCM), and its use as a treatment modality has stood the test of time over thousands of years. Many types of Foot Reflexology, ancient and modern, have been devised and practiced over this time.

Since the advent of the original foot zonal therapy of Dr. Fitzgerald and Eunice Ingham in America, other forms of reflexology have evolved. Some of them encompass zone therapy; others use the Chinese meridian system, the organic system and some use a total energetic concept (such as Light Touch Reflextherapy). There are also several schools of thought as to how much pressure to use – these range from heavy pressure to hardly touching at all – even working in the aura of the foot. Reflected points and pathways are always tender when treatment is required. They are the patient's way of telling the therapist that an imbalance exists in another part of the body. Reflexes must be respected and not be abused in any way.

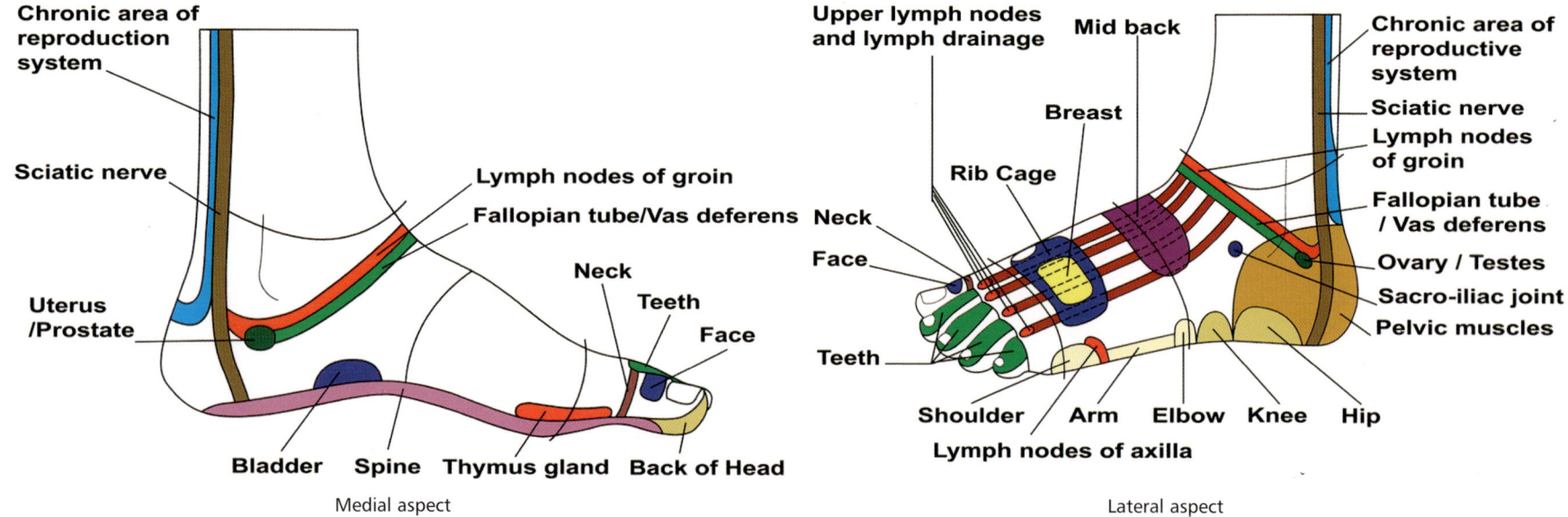

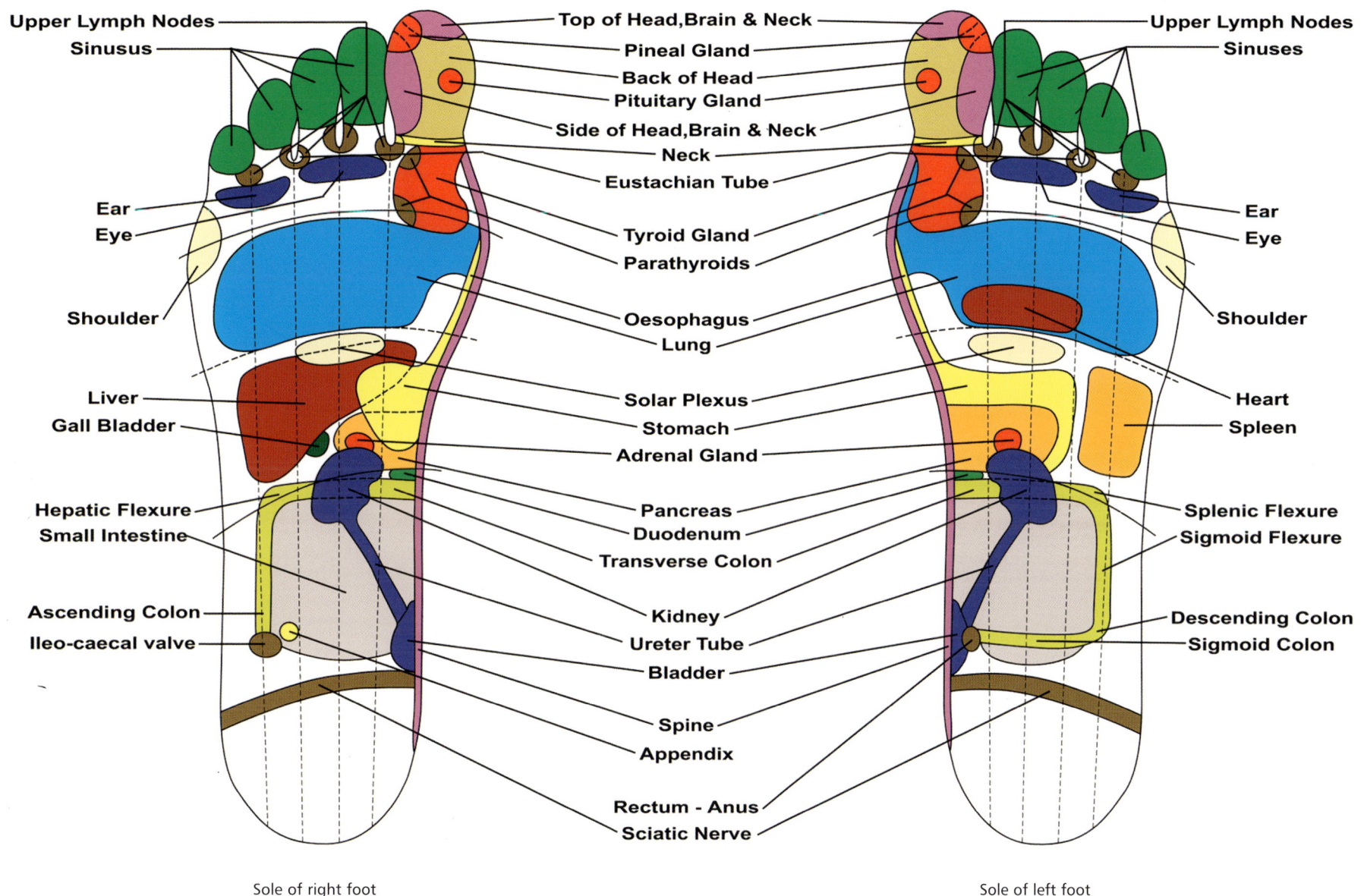

Foot and Leg Meridians

Meridians are the 'energy pathways' in Traditional Chinese and Japanese Medicine' (TCM and TJM) that house and transport 'chi' energy (Vital Force) around the body. Each internal organ has two bilateral associated meridians. There are 12 main organ meridians plus 8 extra-ordinary meridians. Of these, 2 are unilateral (Conception and Governor) and 6 are composites of the original 12. Of the 12 organ meridians, 6 are associated with 'yang' organs – hollow, peristaltic and not essential to life, and 6 are associated with 'yin' organs which are deeper and essential to life.

The 6 meridians (3 Yang and 3 Yin) that are found on the foot and leg are:

Yang – Stomach – Gall Bladder – Bladder
Yin – Spleen – Liver – Kidney

The 3 Yin meridians commence at the Tsing point (by the nail bed) of the toes and travel upwards on the antero-medial aspect of the foot and leg. KI 1 is the only meridian acupoint found on the sole of the foot. The 3 Yang meridians travel down the leg on the postero-lateral aspect and end at the Tsing point. On each meridian, a point called the Great point is highlighted. This is *the* point on the meridian that is probably the most powerful and far reaching in its actions. It is generally the Great point that may be used in combination with either Foot or Hand reflexology to give a more rounded treatment approach.

They are ST 36; GB 42; BL 62; SP 6; LR 3 and KI 6.

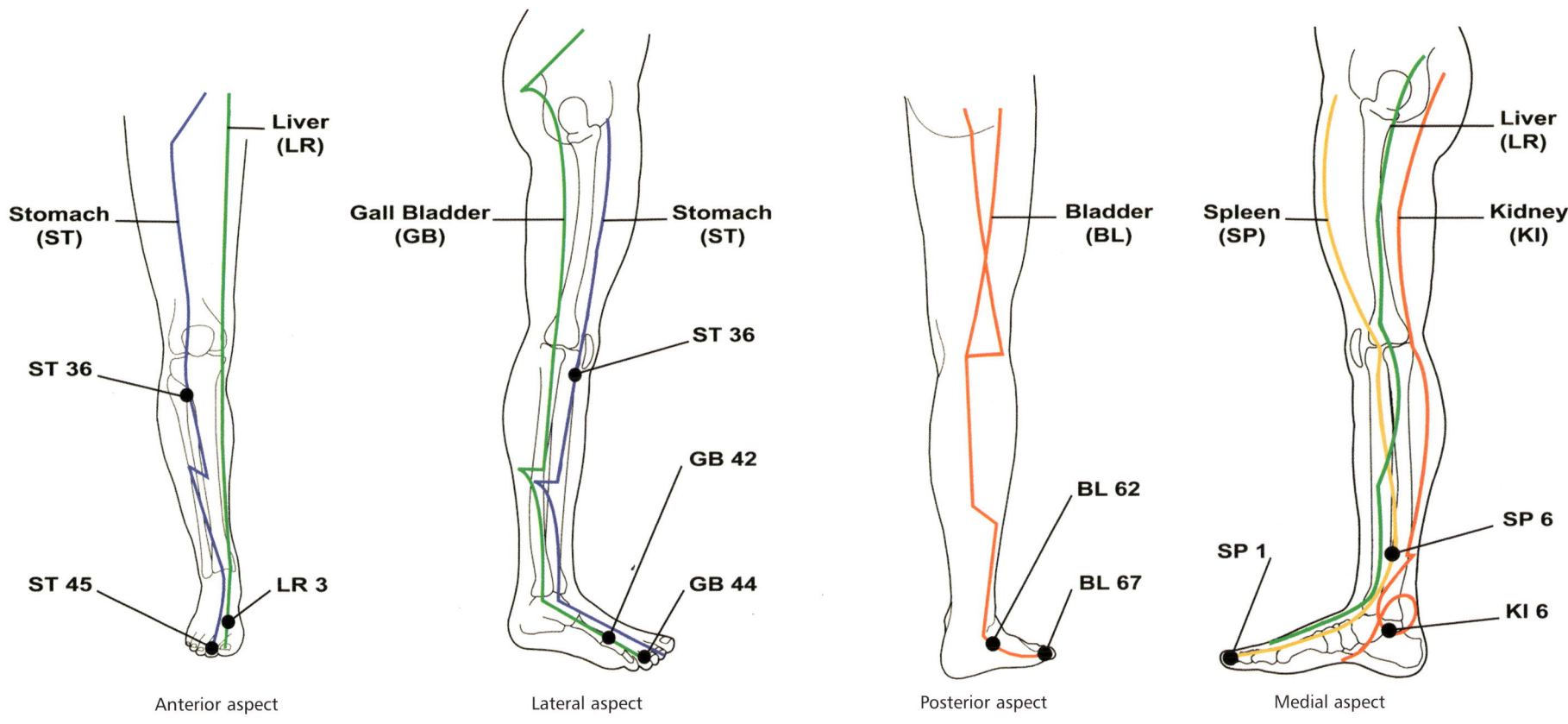

Hand Reflexes

There are several types of reflexes on the hand. The diagrams on the opposite page represent a composite of the reflexes that are used in hand reflexology. This art is much underrated as to its efficacy and had generally taken a back seat compared to its more popular cousin, foot reflexology. Recently, however, it has been discovered and is now being taught at most mainstream reflexology schools.

As stated earlier, in foot reflexology, points and areas requiring treatment exhibit tenderness. Hand reflexes are also tender when intervention is needed, but not in the same 'sharp and acute' way as the foot reflexes. The great beauty of hand reflexology is in the use of self-treatment. It is far easier to teach a patient/client how to massage specific points and areas on his/her hands than for them to massage their feet.

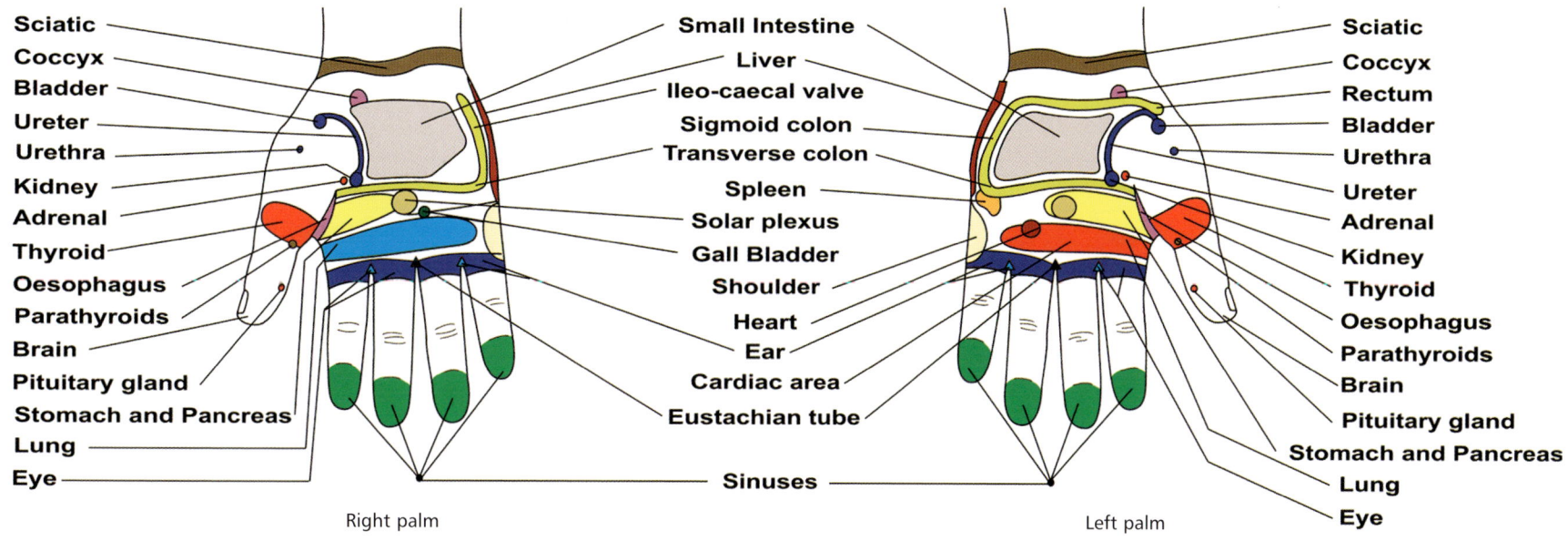

Right palm

Left palm

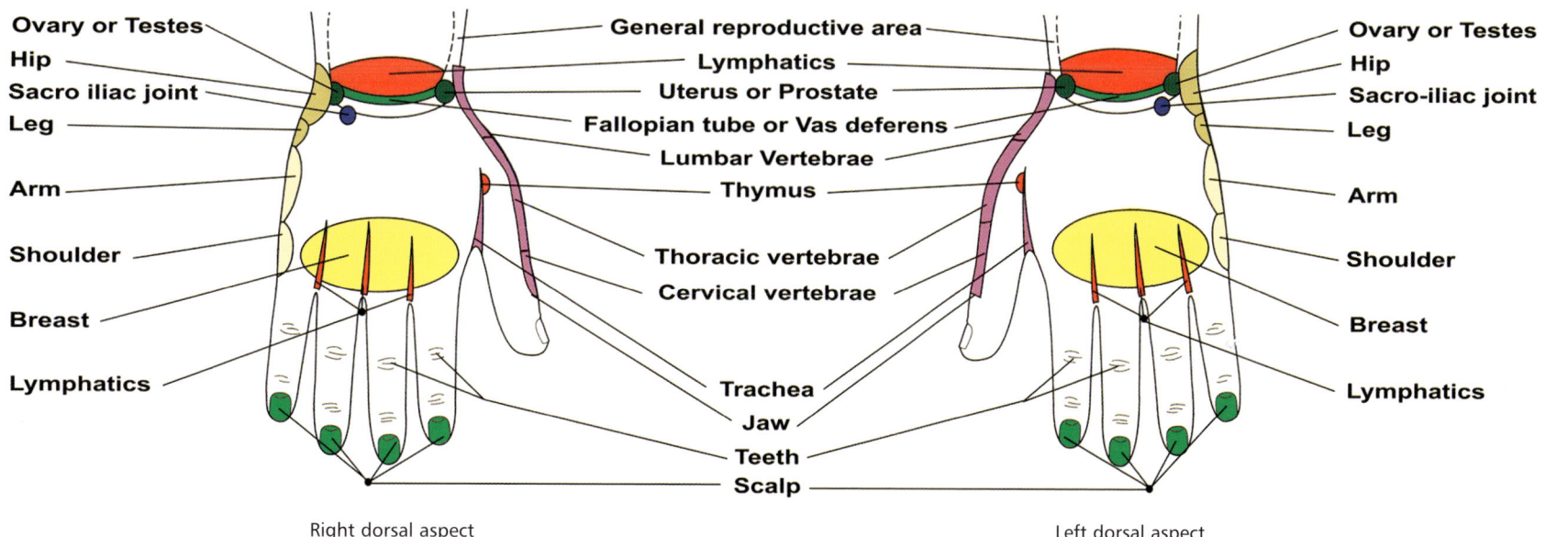

Right dorsal aspect

Left dorsal aspect

Hand Reflexes
Acute Conditions

The reflex points illustrated on the opposite page are based on traditional Japanese and Chinese charts. These points may be used for both analysis and treatment of acute conditions. Like the other reflected points on the body, with a few exceptions, the periphery of the body is represented on the dorsum of the hand and the internal organs are represented on the palmar aspect. Some of the reflex points are also meridian points, e.g. point 2 is also SI 3 and point 15 is also TE 3. Other points are extra meridian points as used in TCM.

In analysis mode, the point should be pressed and gently massaged for just a couple of seconds in order to evoke a response or not. If the response is positive (thus showing that the associated body part requires treatment and energy balancing), the reflex should be acutely tender. If there is little response, this shows that treatment is not required.

When using the reflexes in treatment mode, the points should be gently pressed and rubbed (or just held) for anything up to five minutes. The associated organ or body part should feel more relaxed when using this method. This particular aspect of treatment serves as a very good overture in a whole treatment plan prior to treating the cause of the imbalance. Treating the cause of a condition is admirable but it is pointless in the extreme treating the cause without giving the patient/client some kind of relief. The two can go hand in hand.

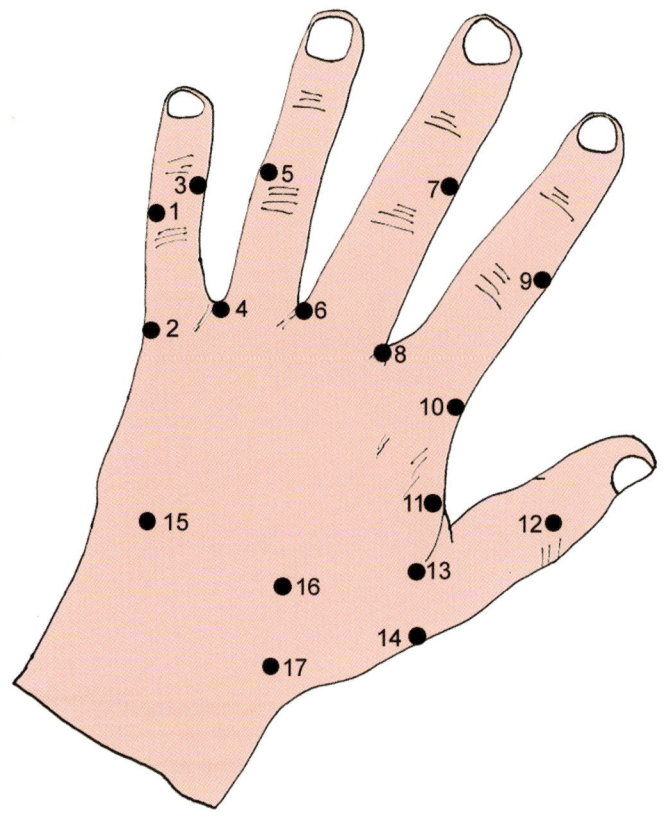

Dorsal aspect

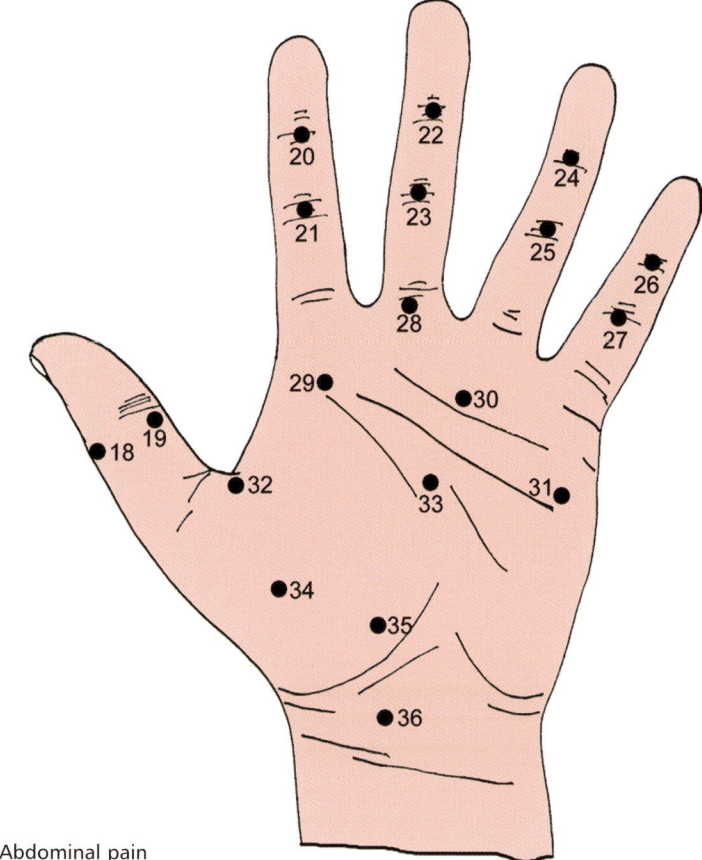

Palmar aspect

INTERNAL ORGANS

1 OCCIPUT Posterior headache
2 VERTEBRAL COLUMN Low back pain
3 PERINEUM Pain in the region
4 SCIATIC NERVE Sciatica, hip pain
5 CRANIUM Pressure headaches
6 THROAT Tonsillitis
7 VERTEX Headache
8 NECK Cervical pain
9 FOREHEAD Frontal Headache
10 SHOULDER Acute painful shoulder
11 NOSE Epistaxis
12 EYE Acute conjunctivitis
13 HEAD Headache
14 ANKLE Sprain or arthritic pain
15 CHEST Intercostal neuritis
16 LEG Sciatica and low back pain
17 SINUSES Sinusitis
18 CHEST Acute asthma

19 G.I. TRACT Abdominal pain
20 LARGE INTESTINE Pain
21 SMALL INTESTINE Diarrhoea
22 HEART Palpitation
23 LYMPHATIC DISORDERS
24 SPLEEN Blood disease
25 LIVER Jaundice
26 KIDNEY Pain
27 BLADDER Cystitis
28 LUNG Chronic coughing
29 THROAT Sore, bronchitis
30 MOUTH Toothache
31 PALPITATION Dizziness
32 HYSTERIA Emotional disturbance
33 EXCESSIVE SWEATING
34 EXCESSIVE COLD Rhinitis
35 STOMACH Pain, vomiting
36 HEEL Sprained ankle

Hand and Arm Meridians

The six meridians that are found on the hand and arm are as follows:

Yin – Lung – Heart – Pericardium
Yang – Large Intestine – Small Intestine – Triple Energiser

The three Yin meridians end at the Tsing (nail) point and are to be found on the antero-medial aspect and the three Yang meridians commence at the Tsing point and are found on the postero-lateral aspect.

The Great points of the six meridians are the most influential in terms of efficacy. They are LU 7; HT 7; PC 6; LI 4; SI 3 and TE 5. They may be used in conjunction with many reflex points, including those of the foot and hand, to enhance treatment.

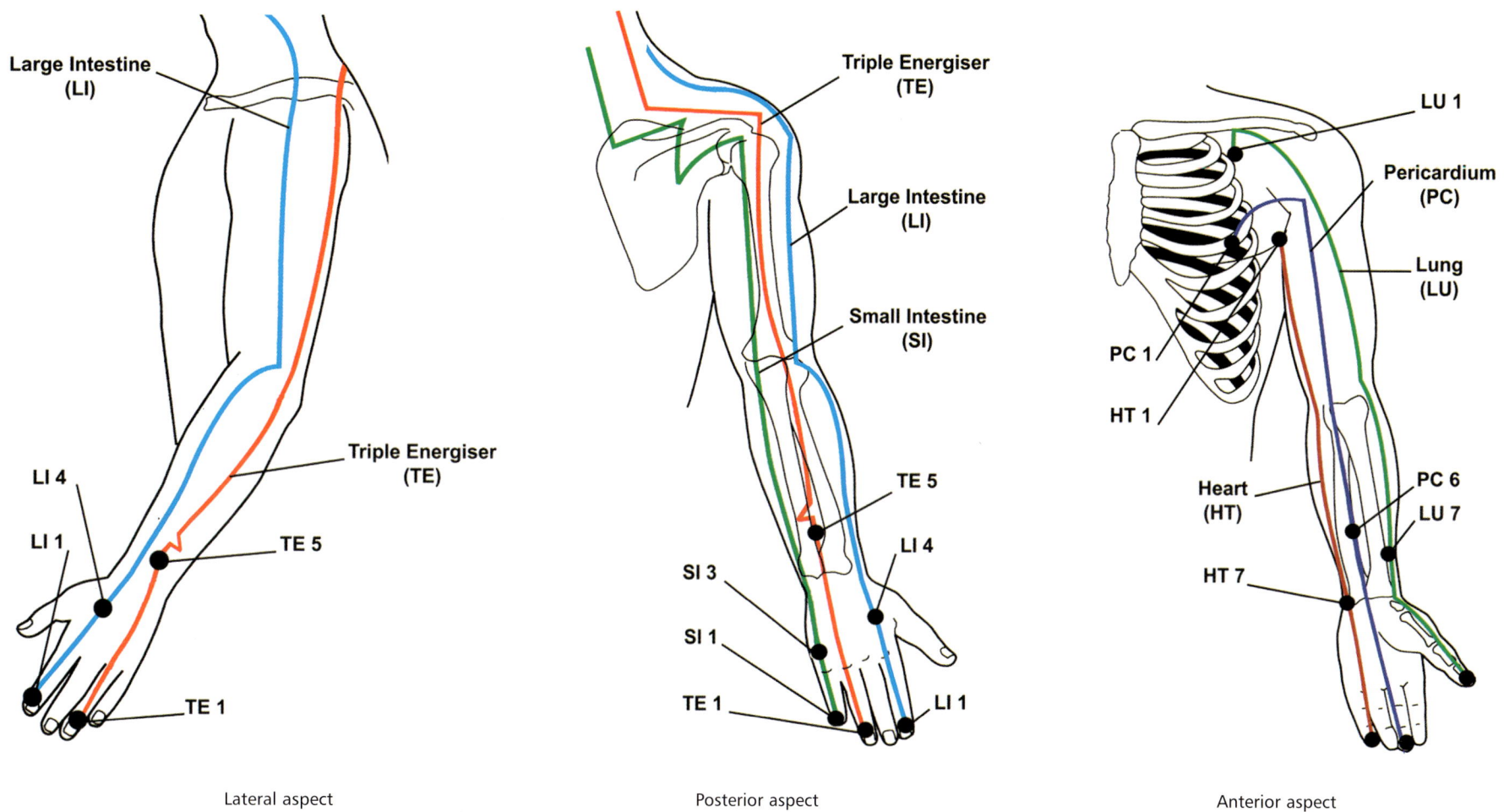

Meridian End Points

The end points of each meridian are very important in both energy analysis and treatment. Each of the end points forms the junction between two different meridians because TCM tells us that the 12 main meridians may be considered as being one long meridian, and it is at the end points that the energy is continued to the next meridian via internal pathways.

The one meridian is: **Stomach** meridian – from eye to 2nd toe to **Spleen** meridian – from great toe to 6th intercostal space to **Heart** meridian – from axilla to little finger to **Small Intestine** meridian from little finger to ear to **Bladder** meridian – from eye to little toe to **Kidney** meridian – from sole of foot to clavicle to **Pericardium** meridian – from chest to middle finger to **Triple Energiser** meridian – from ring finger to ear to **Gall Bladder** meridian – from eye to 4th toe to Liver meridian – from great toe to chest to **Lung** meridian – from chest to thumb to **Large Intestine** – from index finger to nose to **Stomach** meridian, etc.

This workbook cannot explain everything that may be achieved by working with the end points. Two examples are:

1. Using the Tsing (nail) points. Gently palpate each of the Tsing points and give a short clockwise massage to each. Each of the acupoints, being a reflected point of an organ or system, should exhibit some degree of tenderness when palpated. If the patient/client feels acute discomfort to the point of it being uncomfortable, this indicates there is normality or even too much energy in the meridian. If there is no response at all, this indicates that there is very little energy in the meridian and it needs to be stimulated.

2. You may energy balance the meridian between the two end points by placing the middle pad of one middle finger on one end point and the middle pad of the other hand on the other end point. This should be held for up to a couple of minutes. **Please note that the Stomach and Bladder meridians should be held on the second point, as the first point is too close to the eye.**

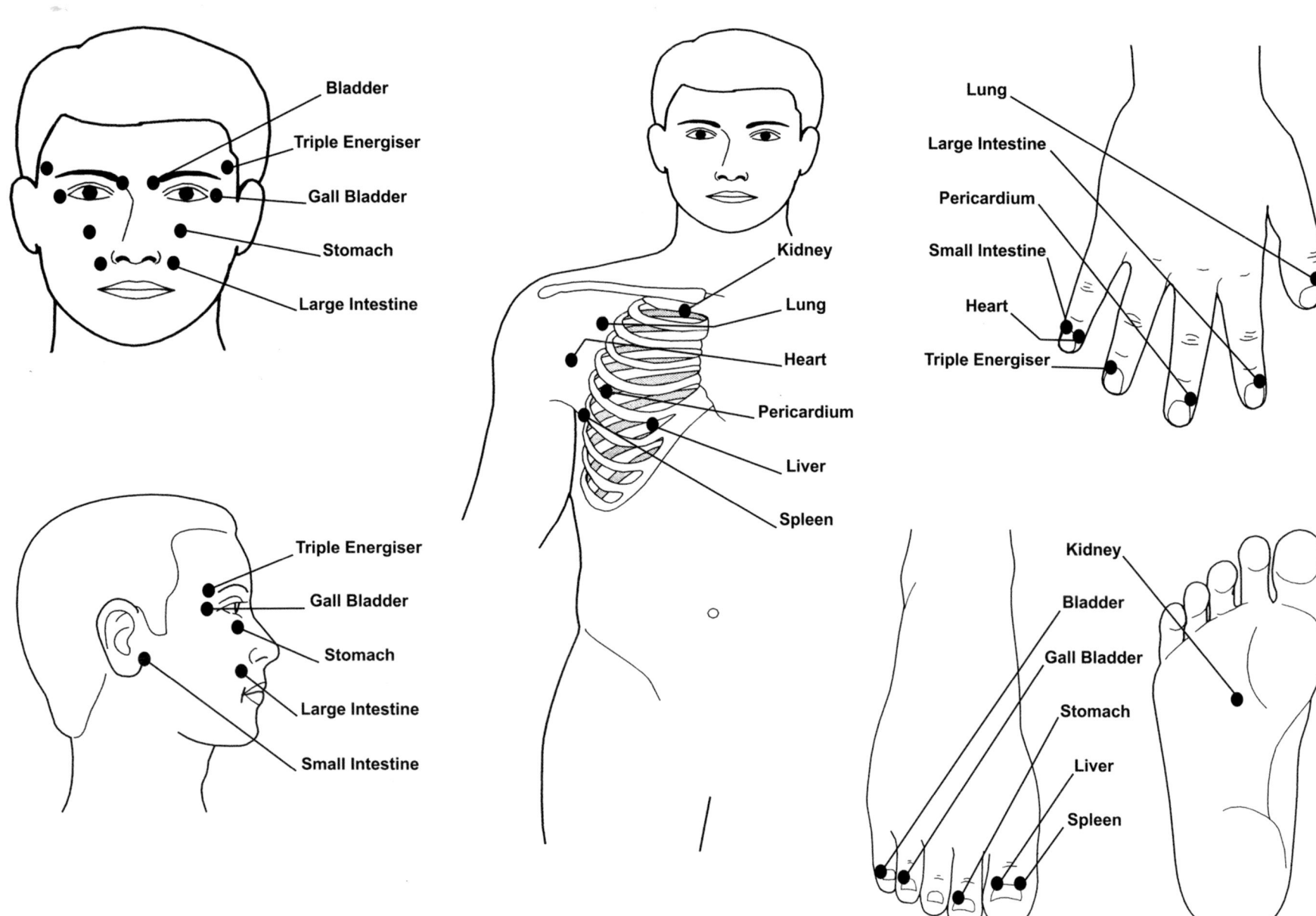

Abdominal Reflex Areas, Alarm Points and Abdominal Meridians

Abdominal Reflex Areas
The abdomen may be divided into reflected areas that correspond with their associated organs. The diagram on the opposite page is a composite of many popular illustrations on the subject. If you press the associated area with a gentle touch and elicit pain or discomfort in the area, this usually indicates an acute inflammatory state in the associated organ. Pain and discomfort found with a deeper palpation indicates a more chronic and long-standing condition. They are sometimes called 'hara' areas. The colours indicate the Five Elements association (see page 48)

Alarm Points
These are often called the 'front' collecting points or 'mu' points. They represent acutely painful 'trigger' spots when the associated organ is in a state of acute imbalance. They may be used in both analysis and treatment. If the point is very acute, it may be energy balanced with another reflected point of that particular organ or with the great point of the meridian.

The hara and alarm points are excellent energy indicators as well as useful treatment tools.

Abdominal Meridians
These are the Conception (Ren Mo), Kidney, Stomach, Liver, Spleen, Gall Bladder and Liver. The energy direction of the Yin meridians (Conception, Kidney, Liver and Spleen) is upwards and the Yang meridians of the Gall Bladder and Stomach downwards.

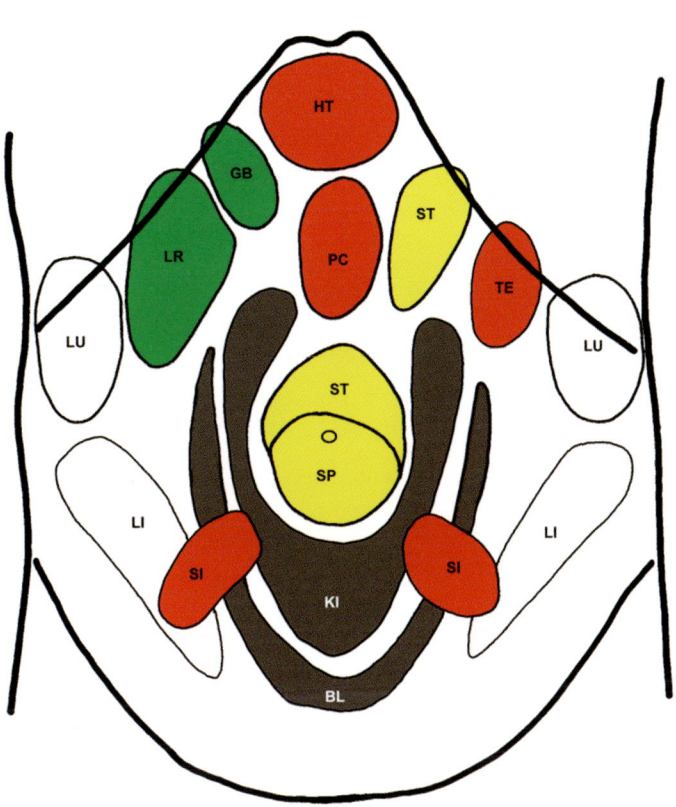

PC	Pericardium	KI	Kidney
HT	Heart	BL	Bladder
SI	Small Intestine	ST	Stomach
TE	Triple Energiser	SP	Spleen
LU	Lung	LR	Liver
LI	Large Intestine	GB	Gall Bladder

Abdominal reflex areas

Alarm points

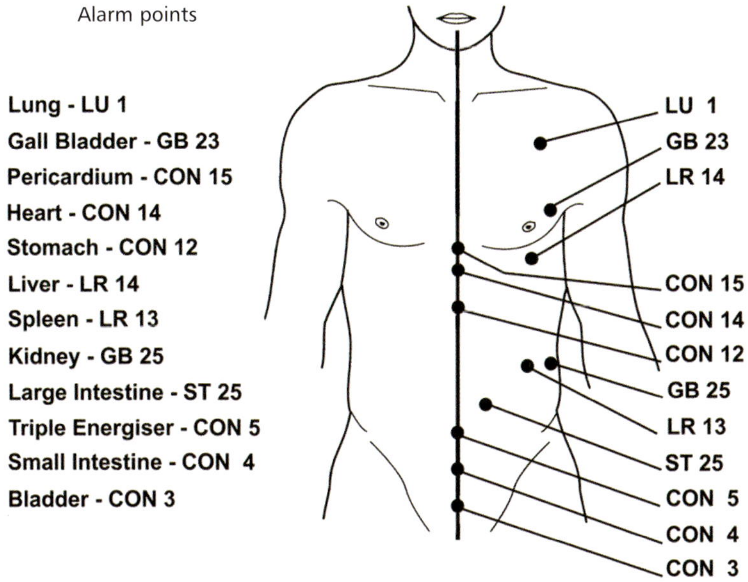

Lung - LU 1
Gall Bladder - GB 23
Pericardium - CON 15
Heart - CON 14
Stomach - CON 12
Liver - LR 14
Spleen - LR 13
Kidney - GB 25
Large Intestine - ST 25
Triple Energiser - CON 5
Small Intestine - CON 4
Bladder - CON 3

Abdominal meridians

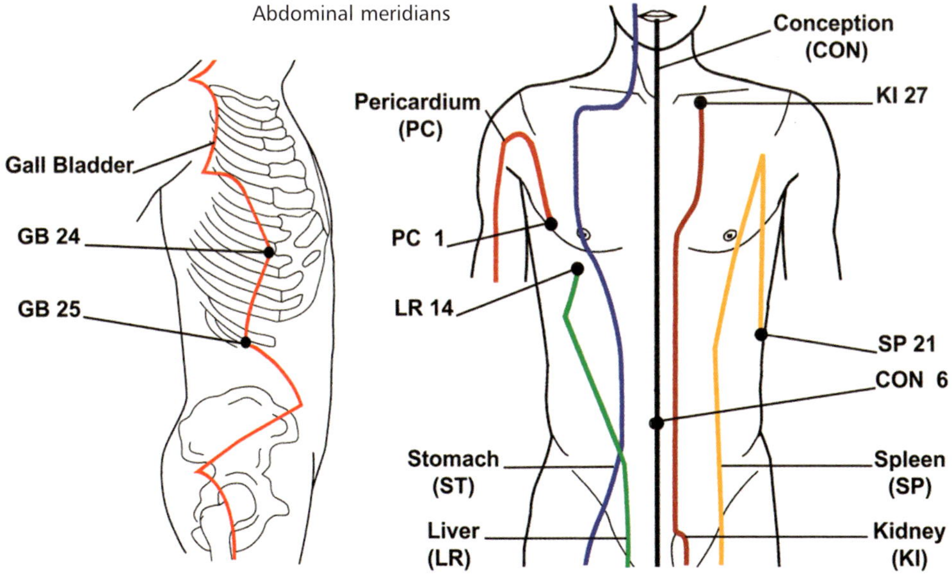

21

Posterior Trunk Meridians and Spinal Zone Reflexes

Posterior Trunk Meridians
These consist of the Governor, Bladder, Small Intestine and a small section of the Gall Bladder. These four meridians are 'yang' in nature with the energy flow of the Governor being upwards and the other three downwards in direction.

Spinal Zone Reflexes
As used in Cranio-sacral Reflexology (CSR)©, these are based upon a combination of different ideas such as the so-called 'Lovett Brother' relationship of the vertebrae, Zone therapy and Occipito-sacral therapy. The five vertical and horizontal zonal regions of the spine, occiput and sacrum are associated with each other. There are many ways of using CSR.

- A tender point on gentle palpation of the nuchal line of the occiput or the upper border of the sacrum will inform you that the corresponding vertebra needs treatment.

- A tender point on the lateral aspect of the sacrum indicates the corresponding vertebra requires treatment and that there may be imbalance of the internal organs associated with that particular vertebra.

For a more comprehensive guide to CSR, see *Acupressure Clinical Applications in Musculo-skeletal Conditions* (Cross, J. R., 2000).

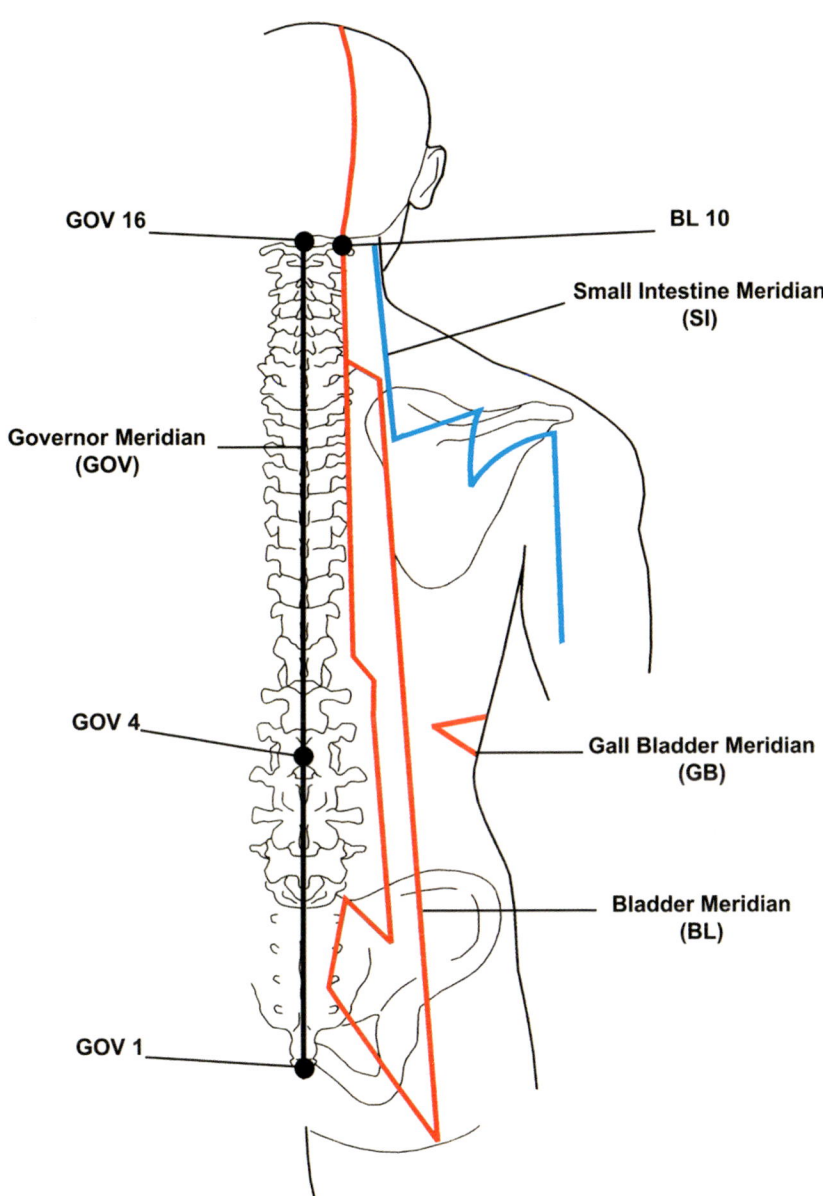

Posterior trunk meridians

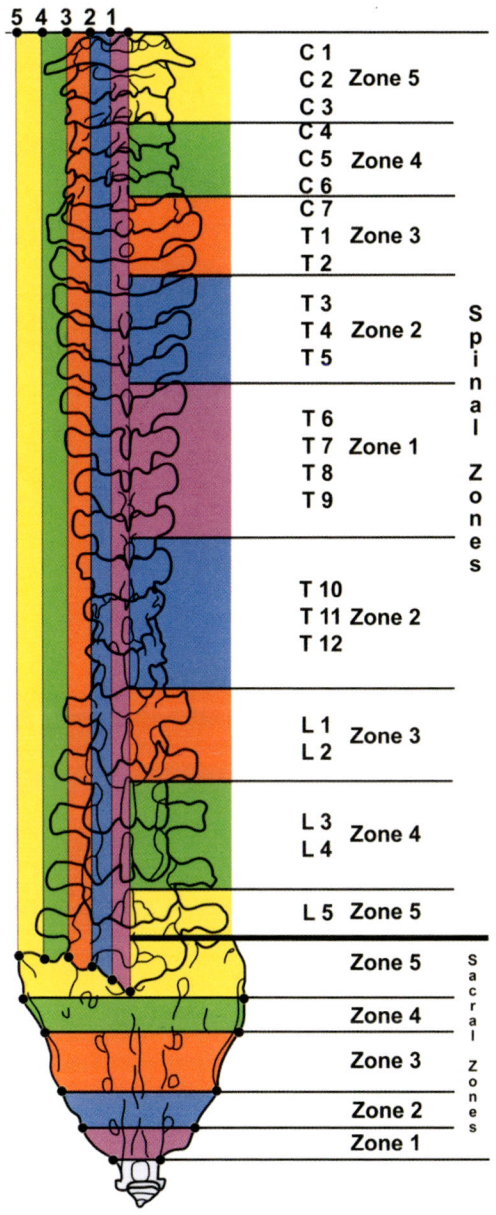

Cranio-sacral reflexology (CSR)

Back Transporting Points and Posterior Trunk Reflexes

Back Transporting Points
These points represent those acupoints situated on the inner bladder meridians (bilaterally) where the associated internal organs may be influenced. This philosophy is part of Traditional Chinese Medicine. Acupuncture is often the preferred therapy but acupressure is very successful especially in the treatment of chronic energy imbalance. An example of how to use these reflexes would be to massage BL 13 (bilateral points) where there is any tightness or congestion in the lungs.

Organ Reflexes
These organ reflexes on the back are the posterior trunk's equivalent of the abdominal reflexes. They may be used in both analysis and treatment and may be extremely useful in the treatment of acute conditions. The colours used indicate the Five Element relationships (see page 48 for an explanation).

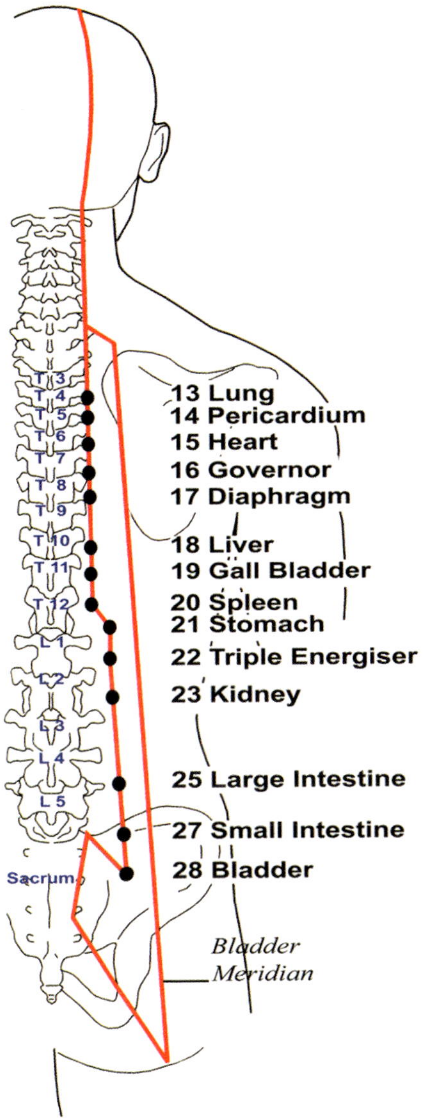

Back transporting points

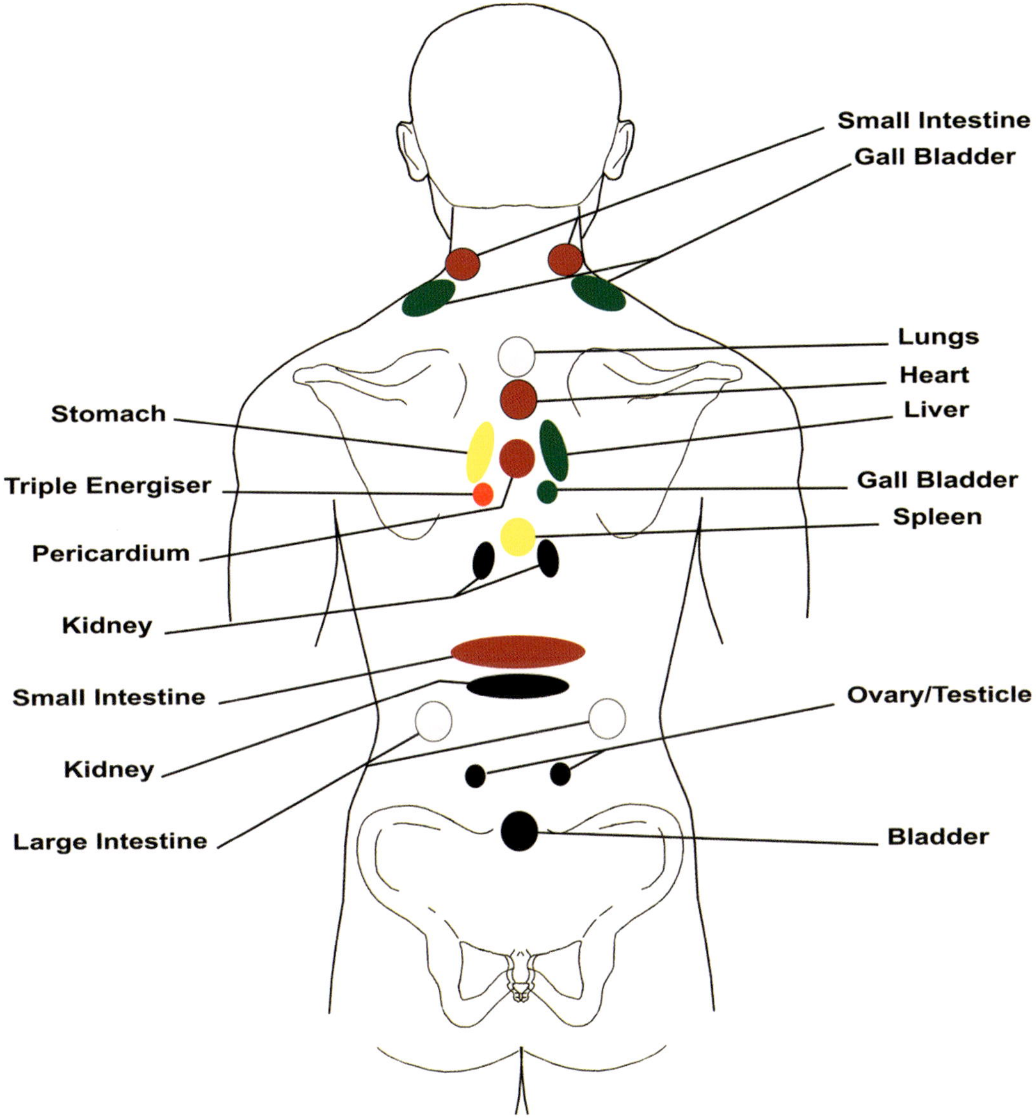

Posterior trunk reflexes

Eye Reflexes
Iris Diagnosis

Iris diagnosis (iridology) represents a fascinating study and one that can take several years to perfect. As with all the reflected pathways in the body, the centre of the iris represents the centre of the body and the outside represents the exterior, i.e. the area just around the pupil represents the stomach and the very outside represents the skin. Just further out from the stomach 'ring' are the small intestine and large intestine. Any irregularity with these organs, such as allergic syndromes or inflammation, shows up as yellow or orange in the form of a 'corona'.

The remainder of the iris represents the rest of the body which may be easily identified by looking at the relevant positions of the hands of the clock. Brown, blue, black or grey markings in the exact area corresponding to an individual body part signifies some state of imbalance in that area of the body. This ranges from acute to chronic imbalances. The spots will disappear following correct and successful treatment.

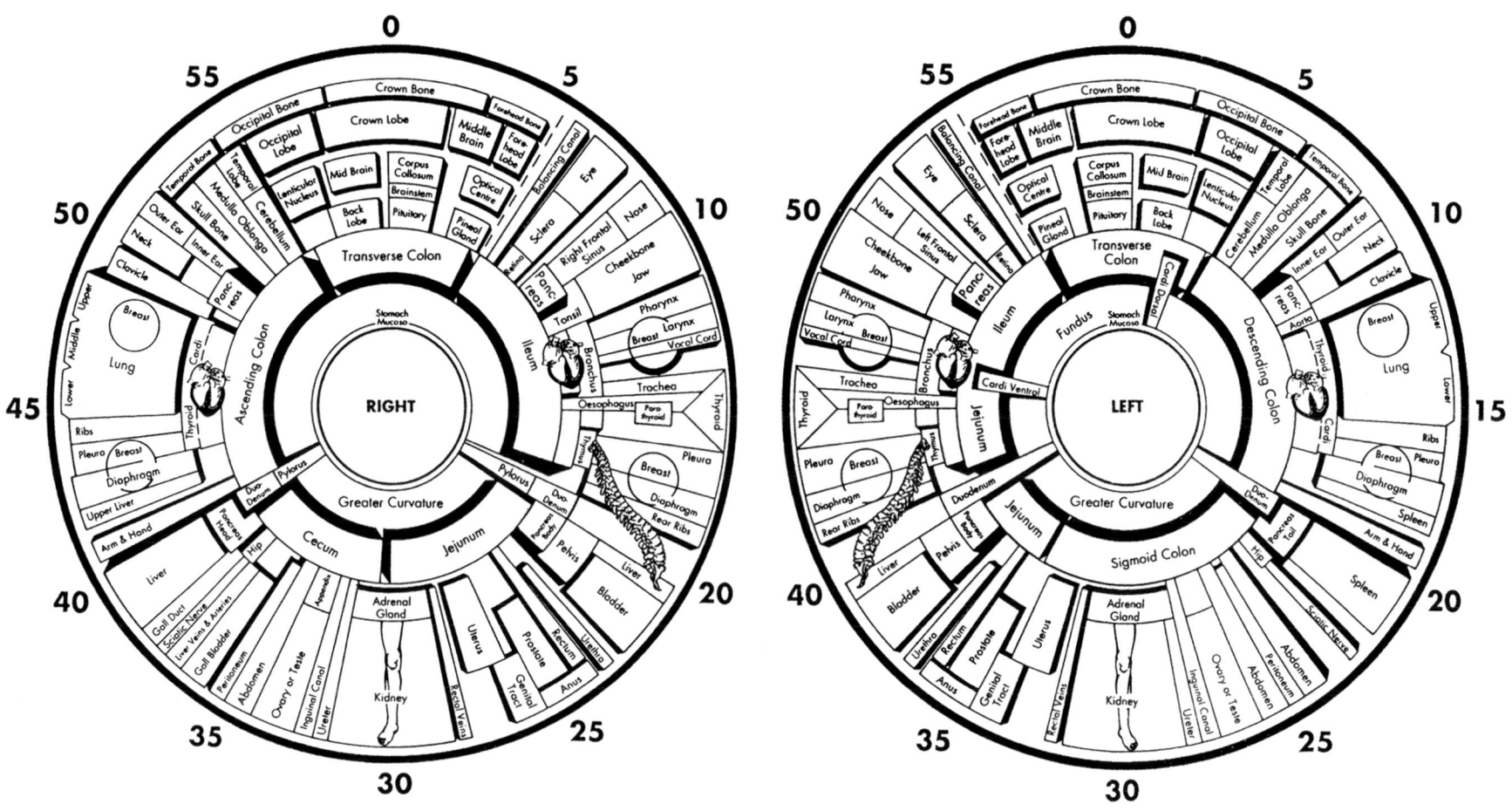

Ear Reflexes
Auriculotherapy

The study of the ear for diagnostic and treatment purposes is a fascinating one that can occupy your mind and brain for several years in order to attain true knowledge. It is again based upon the theory of reflected pathways, in that one can map out the whole of the body within the ear – the centre representing the stomach and the periphery representing the peripheral joints. It is so powerful in acupuncture that I know of several acupuncturists who only use auriculotherapy.

The ear points have diverse uses. They are extremely useful in analgesia and the treatment of addiction and allergic responses. You may use the tip of the little finger or a 'baby bud' to affect the corresponding region.

For the treatment of pain, the finger or bud is placed on the reflected area for about 3 minutes – this is particularly helpful in acute discomfort.

Addictions may be helped with auriculotherapy. Depending on the particular addiction, points such as the stomach, liver, lungs, brain stem and 'shen men' may be used. Small seed pellets, magnets or tiny coiled dermal pins may be used in some cases.

Allergies may be helped by leaving a small pin in the liver, shen men and endocrine points.

Please note that extensive training is required to do many of these techniques and treatments should not be undertaken without it.

Ear apex
Heel
Toe
Ankle joint
Ankle
TRIANGULAR FOSSA
Knee joint
Uterus
External genital
Asthma point
Hepatitis point
Sympathetic nerve
Constipation
Thigh joint
Sciatic nerve
Shen-men
Heat point
Knee
Wrist
LOWER CRURA OF ANTIHELIX
Urethra
Urinary bladder
CYMBA CONCHA
Large intestine
Lower rectum
Buttock
Gall bladder
Sacral vertebrae
Kidney
Pancreas
Outer ear
CRUS OF HELIX
ANTERIOR INCISURE
Ear centre
Esophagus
Appendix
Small intestine
Duodenum
Diaphram
Liver
Abdomen
Elbow
Mouth
Stomach
Lower abdomen
Throat
TRAGUS
Pharynx
EXTERNAL AUDITORY MEATUS
CAVUM CONCHA
External nose
Upper abdomen
Adrenal
Internal nose
Bronchus
Spleen
Chest
Trachea
Lung
Heart
Subcortex
Brainstem
Brain point
Pingchuan
Parotid gland
Testis
(ovary)
Temple
Thyroid
Neck
Clavicle
ANTITRAGUS
INTERTRAGIC INCISURE
Eye I
Internal secretion
Eye II
Forehead
Tongue
Lower jowl (mandible)
Upper jowl
Upper teeth
Cheek
LOBULE
Lower teeth
Eye
Internal ear
Tonsil
UPPER CRURA OF ANTIHELIX
Finger
Minor occipital nerve
AURICULAR TUBERCLE
Urticaria
Hip joint
Liver yang
HELIX
Lumbago point
Lumbar vertebrae
SCAPHOID FOSSA
ANTIHELIX
Shoulder
Muscle relax point
Thorax
Mammary gland
Shoulder joint
Thoracic vertebrae
Cervical vertebrae
Soft palate
Occiput
TAIL OF HELIX

Groove for lowering blood pressure
Upper portion of the back
Middle portion of the back
Lower portion of the back

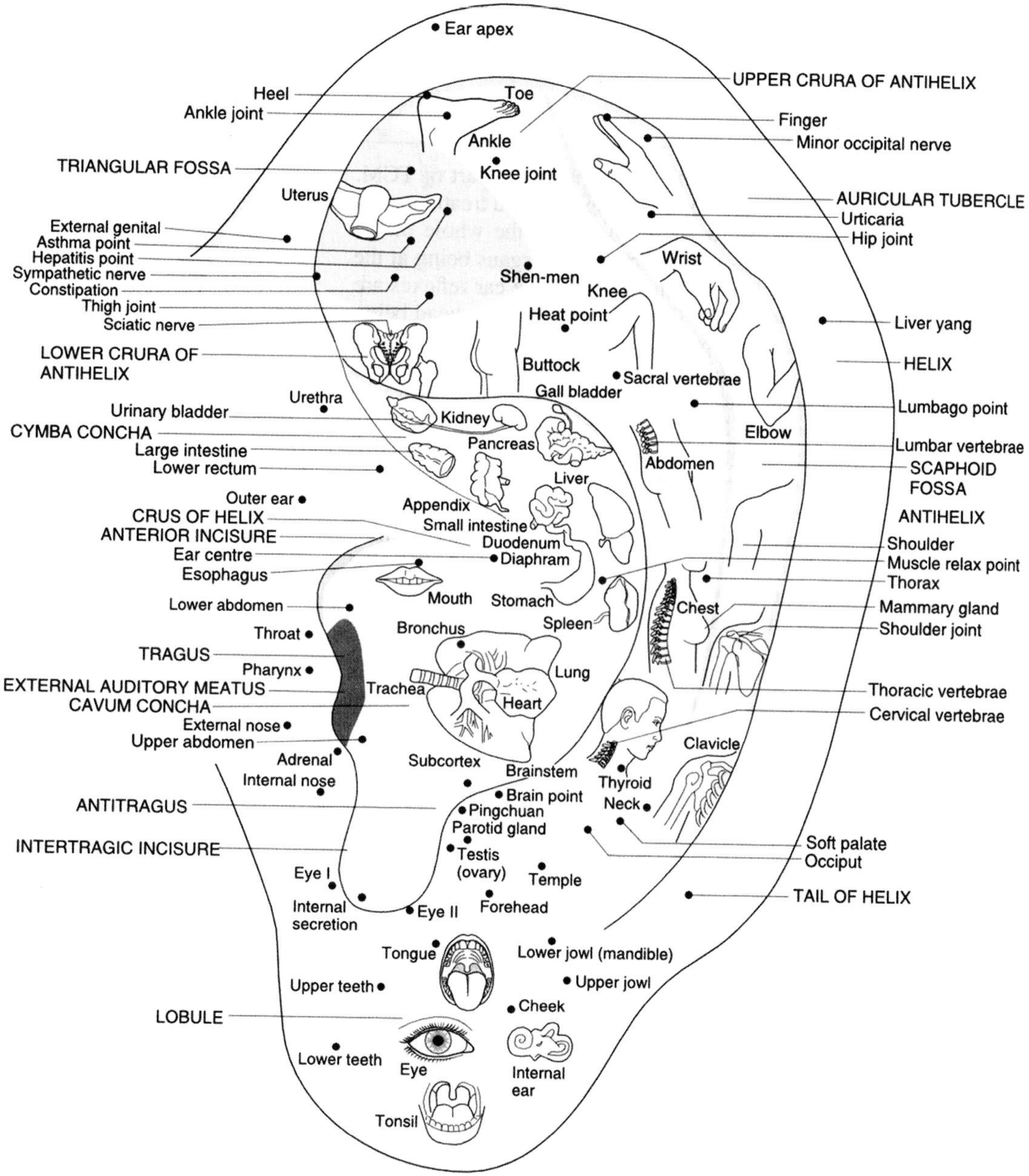

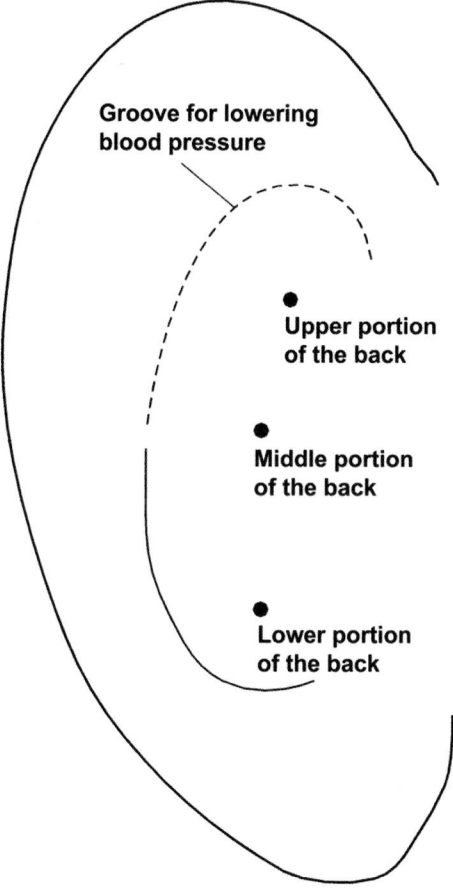

Tongue, Pulse and Teeth Reflexes
Tongue Diagnosis, Pulse Diagnosis and Holistic Dentistry

Tongue Reflexes
The tongue has been a useful analytical tool for centuries and is a major player in TCM. It is said that the tongue represents the outward expression of the stomach and that any imbalance within the digestive system can be detected there. The tongue also represents the reflected areas of the body. It is a most reliable indicator and changes often appear in the tongue prior to physical symptoms. Tongue diagnosis takes many months of study. The colours represent those of the Five Elements (see page 48)

Pulse Reflexes
Pulse diagnosis is one of the oldest of all traditional diagnostic methods. The discerning practitioner may detect six different pulses on the radial artery just superior to the wrist crease. There are three superficial and three deep pulses on each wrist that correspond to the twelve organs. The pulse may be 'full', 'superficial', 'floating', 'slippery', 'choppy' and any one of up to twenty-seven variations. This procedure represents a long study to perfect – sometimes a lifetime!

Teeth Reflexes
Recently, a new paradigm called Holistic Dentistry has come to the fore. It states that each tooth is associated with a particular internal organ and that problems with each tooth may be caused by imbalance with its associated organ. There are several charts available and the one shown on the opposite page represents a composite of these.

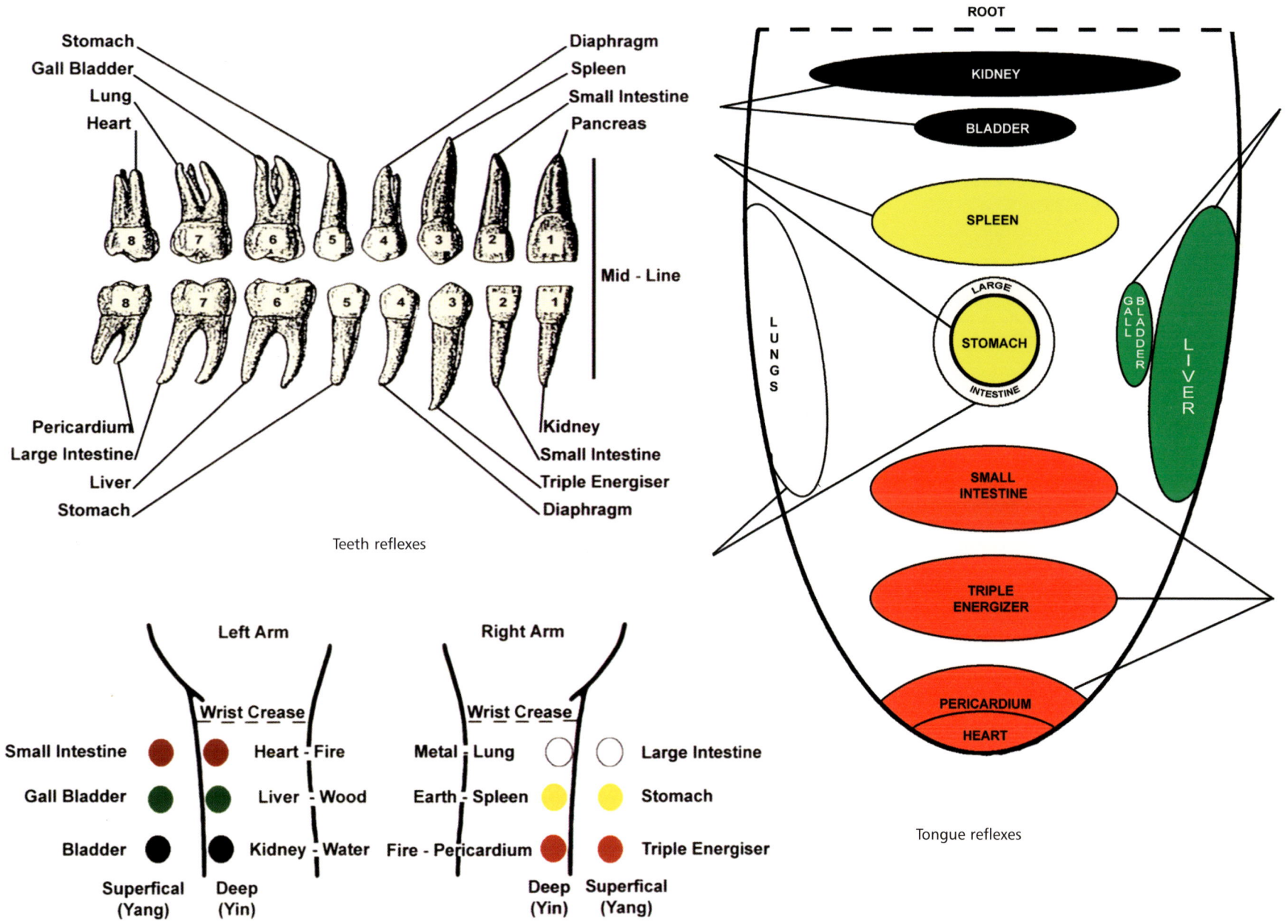

Teeth reflexes

Pulse diagnosis

Tongue reflexes

Facial Reflexes
Facial Diagnostic Areas, Acute and Chronic Reflex Points

Facial Diagnostic Areas
There are several different interpretations of this. They differ according to the traditional philosophy, i.e. Chinese, Japanese or Ayurvedic. The illustration opposite represents those correspondences borne out by personal experience. Although the colours are those of the Five Elements Law (see page 48), the reflected areas do not necessarily show the associated colour when the organ is in a state of energy imbalance – but often it does. An example would be when someone is suffering from a chronic kidney condition; there is a telltale black hue underneath the eyes.

Acute Reflex Points
These reflexes do not relate to individual organs or energy channels as such, but deal with the treatment of acute conditions. Many of the points are the same as meridian acupoints, some are based on old shamanic charts and others are based on Applied Kinesiology. Point 2, for instance, is Gov 20, point 16 is Yintang (Brow chakra) and point 13 is GB 14. These points just need to be held with the finger pad for a few minutes until there is relief of discomfort.

Chronic Reflex Points
This diagram looks more like someone with chickenpox than one of facial reflexes. These reflexes are based on traditional Chinese and Japanese charts and are used solely in the treatment of chronic conditions. They are extremely useful for the client/patient to use themselves, massaging the required point every couple of hours for 2 to 3 minutes.

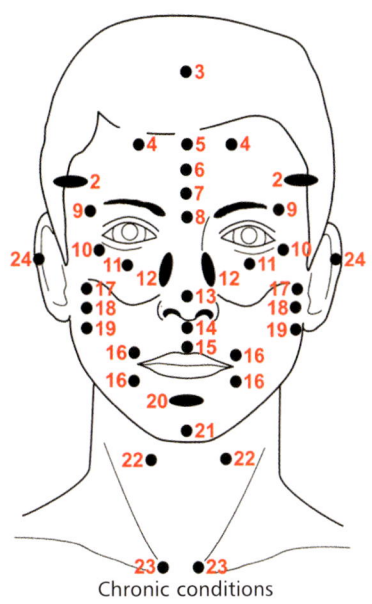
Chronic conditions

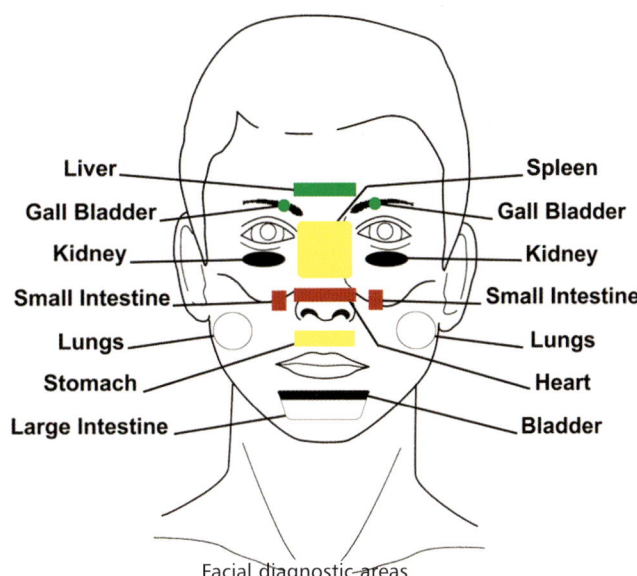
Facial diagnostic areas

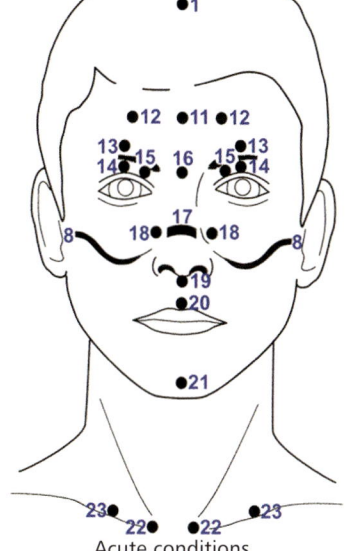
Acute conditions

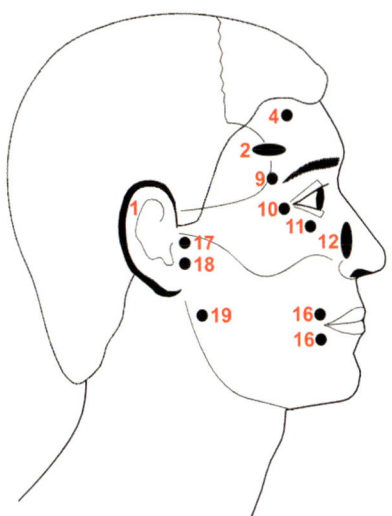

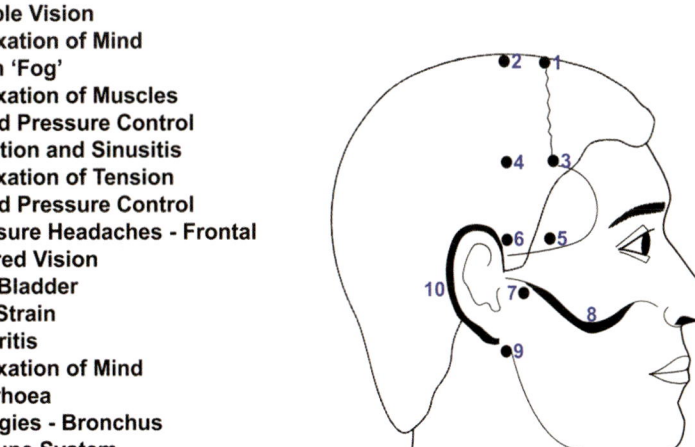

1. Blood Circulation
2. Sciatica
3. Reproductive Organs
4. Memory
5. Autonomic Nervous System
6. Pelvic Region
7. Insomnia
8. Headaches/Eye Strain
9. Stomach
10. Large Intestine
11. Kidney
12. Large and Small Intestine
13. Stomach
14. Spleen
15. Pancreas
16. Lungs
17. Heart
18. Liver and Gall Bladder
19. Lymphatics
20. Bladder
21. Constipation
22. Sexual
23. Thyroid
24. Blood Circulation

1. Pressure Headaches - Top of Head
2. Relaxation of Mind
3. Double Vision
4. Relaxation of Mind
5. Brain 'Fog'
6. Relaxation of Muscles
7. Blood Pressure Control
8. Infection and Sinusitis
9. Relaxation of Tension
10. Blood Pressure Control
11. Pressure Headaches - Frontal
12. Blurred Vision
13. Gall Bladder
14. Eye Strain
15. Gastritis
16. Relaxation of Mind
17. Diarrhoea
18. Allergies - Bronchus
19. Immune System
20. Anti - Sneeze
21. Constipation
22. Thyroid Metabolism
23. Angina and Palpitation

33

Face and Head Meridians

The facial and head meridians shown on the opposite page in anterior and lateral aspects may initially seem a little daunting to learn. The anterior aspect is shown with the bilateral meridians on one side of the face only to allow for clarity. The end points of the meridians are shown with the exception of the Governor which ends on the underside of the top lip.

The meridians are Bladder; Gall Bladder; Stomach; Triple Energiser; Small Intestine; Large Intestine and the unilateral meridians of the Conception and Governor.

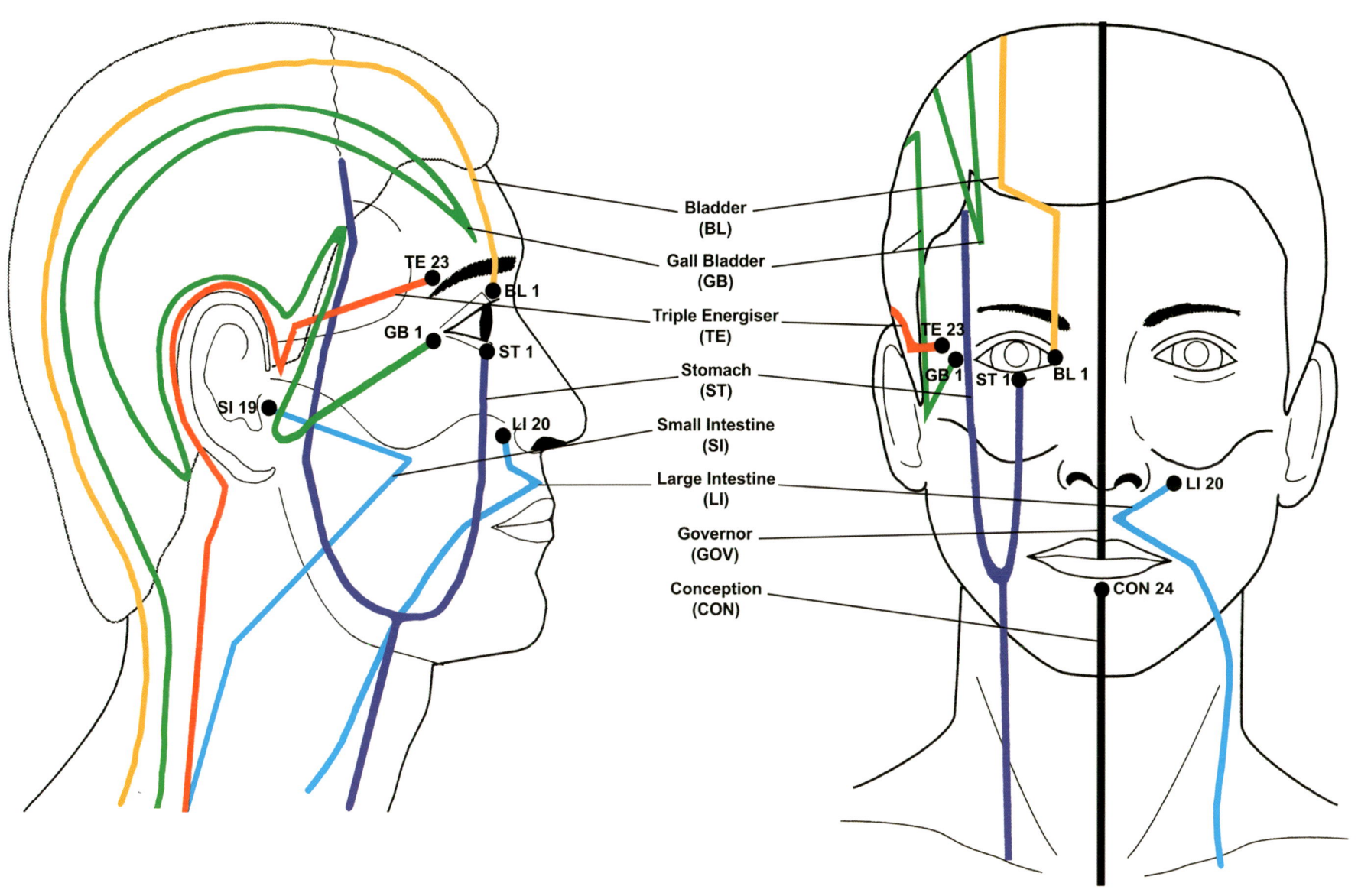

Head Stress Reflexes

These little known reflexes are sometimes called 'stretch' reflexes and are associated with the body's muscles (with the notable exception of the temporo-mandibular joint (TMJ). This approach forms part of the Applied Kinesiology philosophy, which was devised by American chiropractors in the early 1960s. It is a very useful adjunct to treatment.

As with all reflected areas, the whole of the body (in this case muscles) may be mapped out on both the skull and hand. The great strength of these reflexes is in the treatment of chronic muscular imbalance and is often used at the commencement of more general muscular treatment such as deep massage.

Whenever there is muscular weakness – either due to spasm or post surgery (e.g. weak quadriceps following a meniscectomy) – the pads of the opposing fingers should be placed gently on the reflex and simply held there for about half a minute until warmth is felt. A slight stretching movement is then given, very subtly, attempting to part the fingers of each hand from each other but not actually moving the fingers on the patient's skin. This is usually done for about 2 to 3 minutes or until the patient indicates that the corresponding muscle feels 'different'.

Please note that you do not need to be a practitioner of either Applied Kinesiology or 'Touch For Health' to be able to use these reflexes.

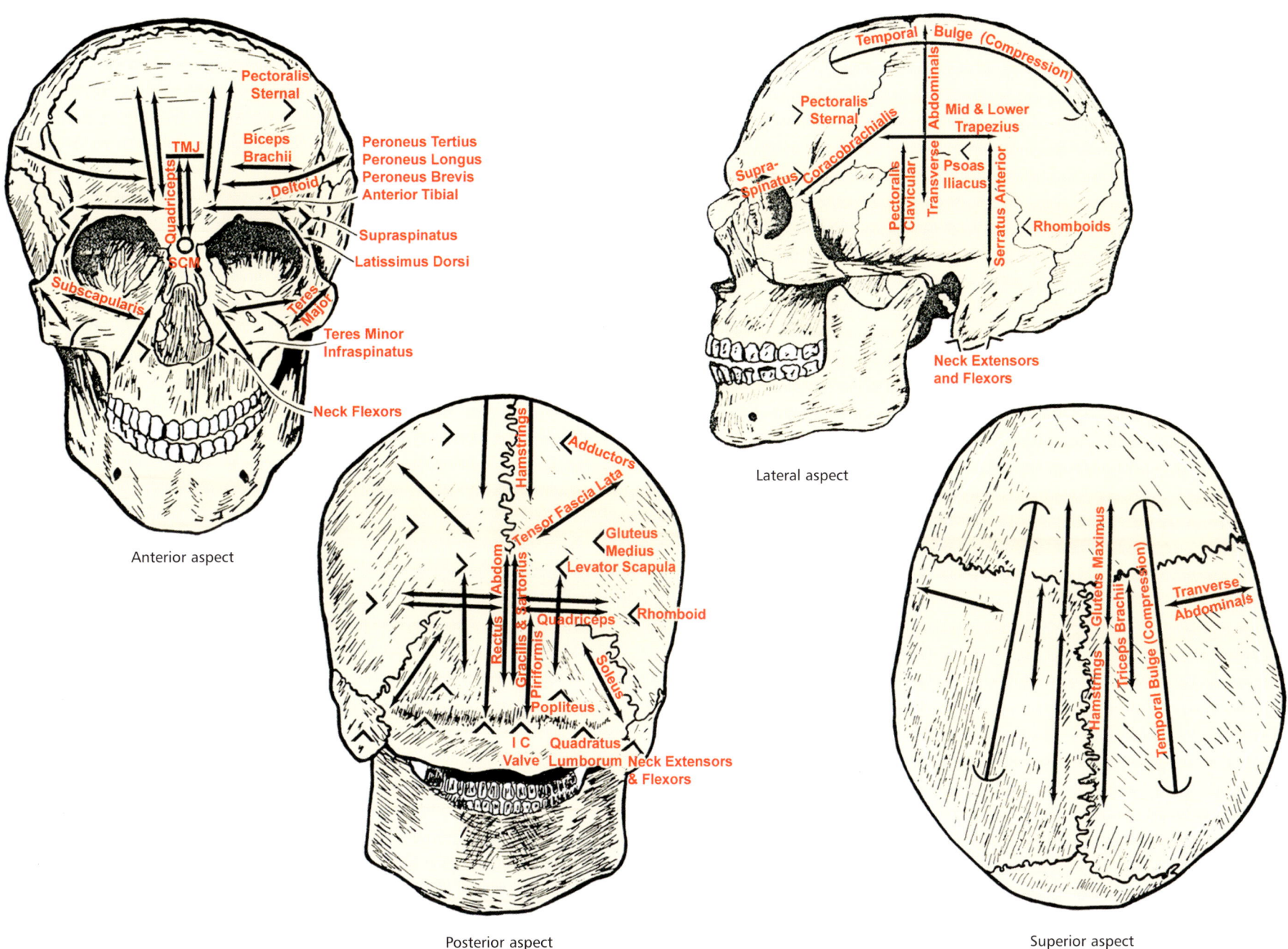

Hand Stress Reflexes

In my opinion, the skull reflexes are more 'powerful' than the hand ones – the latter, though, are ideal tools for the patient to use in self-help. In this scenario, the patient is asked to gently stretch the reflex that is associated with the weak muscle by using the thumb and forefinger in opposition. Imagine someone who is suffering from a painful neck and is experiencing tightness and tension in the trapezius and neck extensor muscles as a consequence of this. Direct therapy on the muscles (massage, etc.) may be too sore for the patient. The answer is to get them to use the Stress Reflexes on the hands a few times a day until the muscles are more receptive to direct treatment.

Please note that a muscle experiencing pain and spasm is a *weak* muscle, not a strong one!

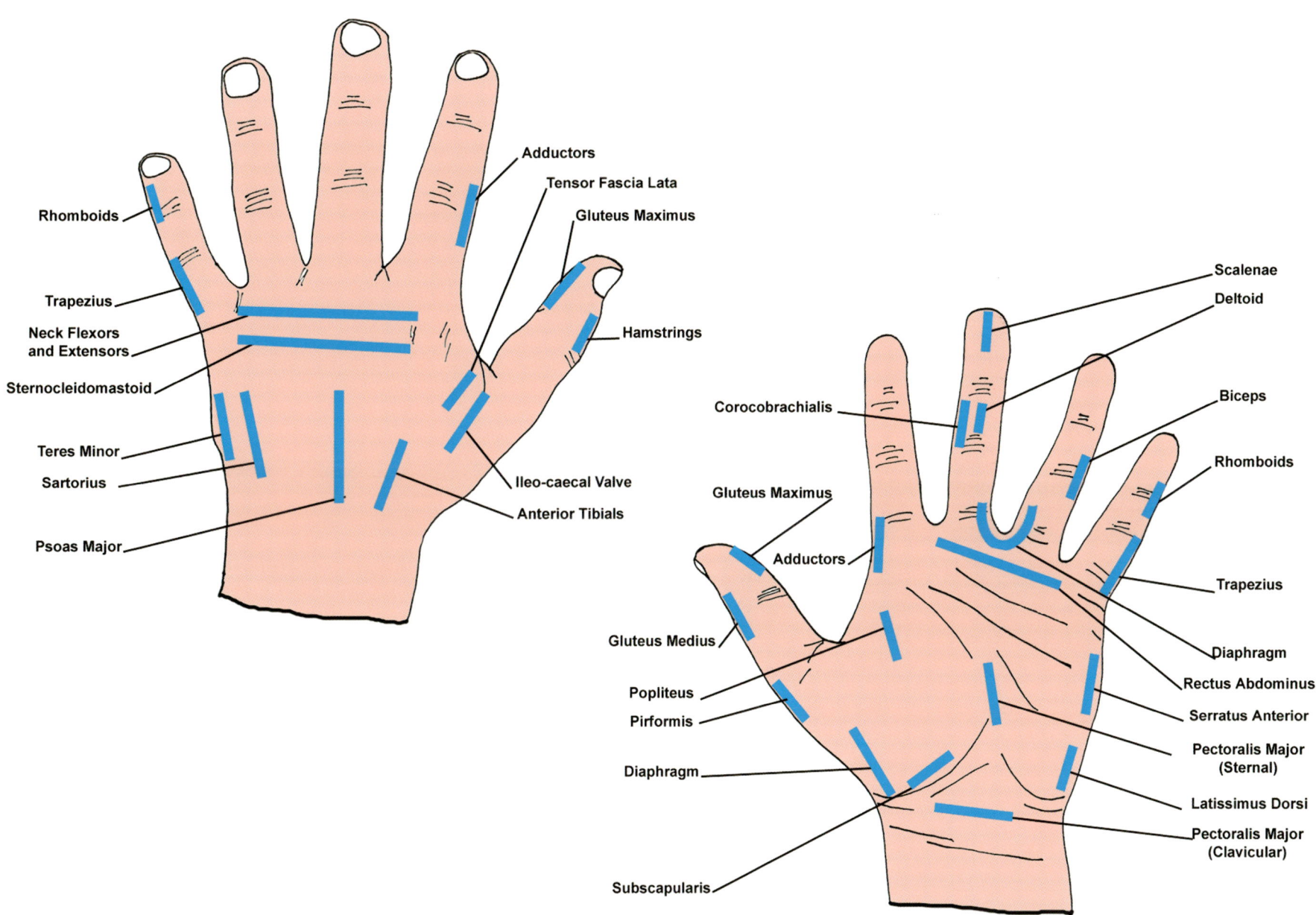

Neurovascular Reflexes on the Head

In the early 1930s, a chiropractor and naturopath called Terence Bennett developed the Bennett reflexes. These reflex points, located around the head, were postulated to affect the circulation of the vascular system of various organs and glands to improve many types of conditions. In 1966, Dr. George Goodheart correlated Bennett's reflexes with the muscle weaknesses found in Applied Kinesiology. He found that stimulating these reflexes could bring strength to a weak muscle.

It is believed that each neurovascular point is placed and obtains its correlation with its associated organs and muscles as the embryo unfolds. The reflex is stimulated by a very light touch, just giving it a slight 'tug' and holding it for about twenty seconds.

These reflexes make an excellent adjunct to treatment, especially in the treatment of musculo-skeletal conditions. They are usually used towards the end of a treatment session.

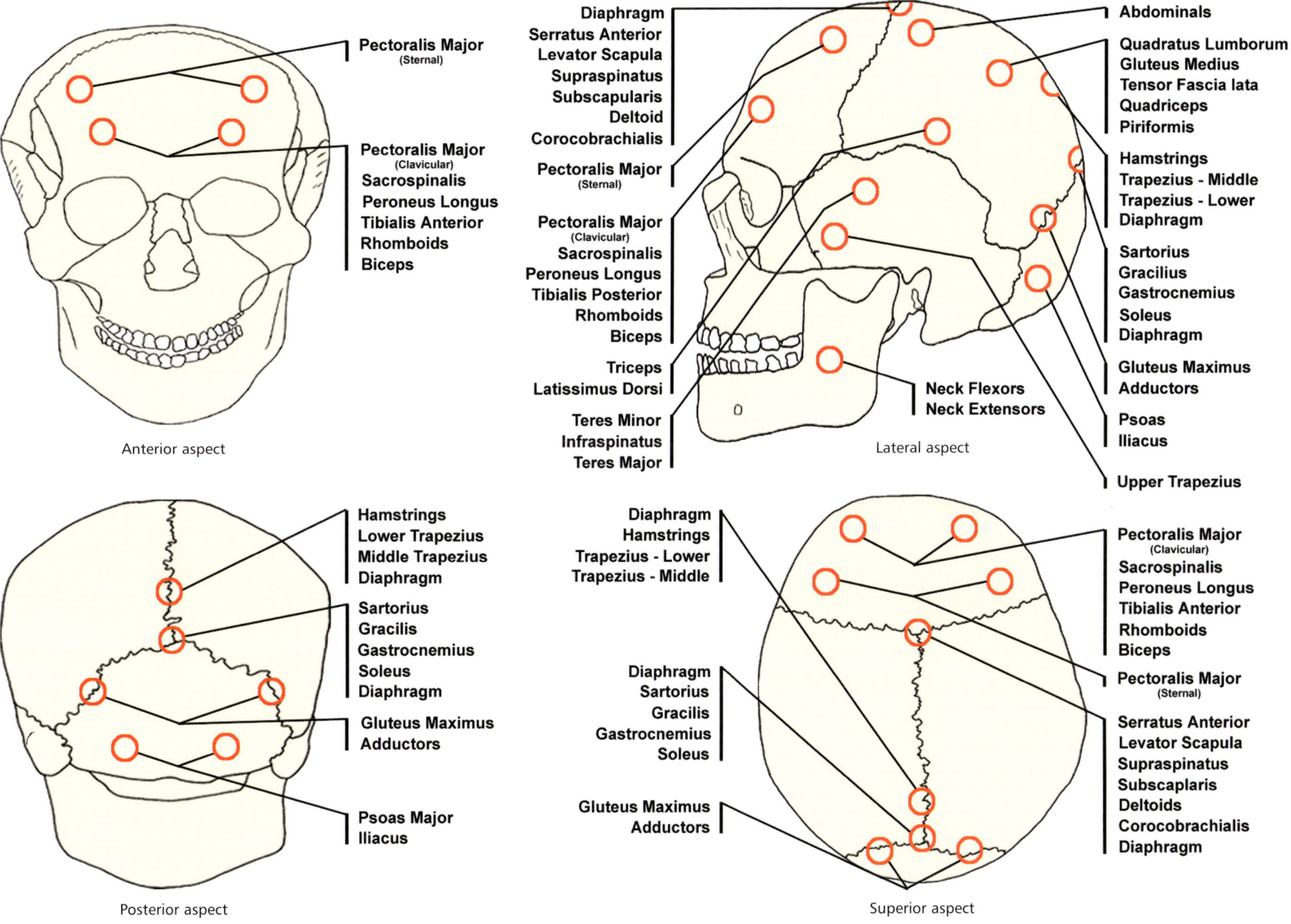

Temporo-sphenoidal Line
Spinal and Muscular Reflexes

The knowledge of the Temporo-sphenoidal Line (TSL) dates back to the pioneer days of the last century with Dr. George Goodheart and other pioneers of Applied Kinesiology. In the original texts it quite categorically stated that the TSL is used in analysis only, but I have modified the theory to include treatment benefits as well. Several points of acute tenderness may exist along the TSL. These points were firstly just associated with individual muscles where it was found that the point was tender when a particular muscle was in a state of energetic imbalance. When I studied this phenomena in the late 1970s, I soon realised that constant muscle testing was not my favourite occupation.

I formulated the TSL to be a powerful reflected region to show the vertebral levels as well. In analytical mode, discomfort on gentle palpation shows imbalance in the corresponding vertebra – acute lesions showing more acute tenderness than chronic lesions. In treatment mode, once the level of spinal lesion is known, the relevant reflex is held either side of the head with the middle finger pads – maybe for as long as five minutes. This affords relief of tension and discomfort at the vertebral level being treated and paves the way for more intensive therapy using local treatment or other reflected points for that particular spinal level.

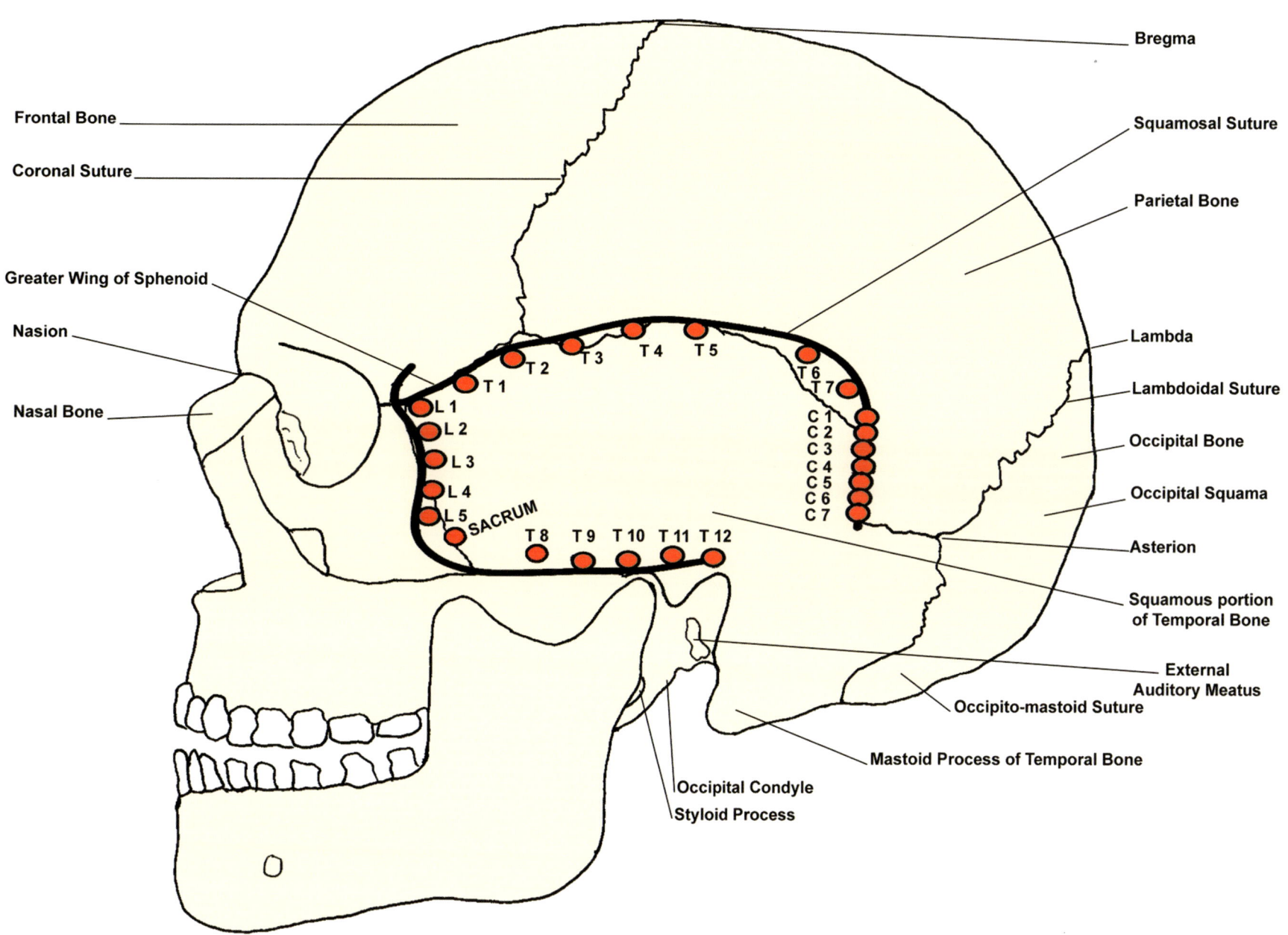

Neurolymphatic Points
Chapman's Reflexes

These important reflexes were 'discovered' by Dr. Frank Chapman, an American osteopath in the 1930s. He found that lymphatic drainage would be stimulated by massaging certain tender points on the body. Modern Applied Kinesiology has taken these reflexes to heart and changed the name to Neurolymphatic points (NL) and given muscular associations to each of the reflex points.

My research into NL points and areas in the early 1980s has placed emphasis on each of the NL points and areas being related to individual meridians which in turn affect the related internal organs. This is the illustration shown on the opposite page.

There are two ways that the NL points may be used in therapy:
1. in isolation to aid a specific organ/meridian,
2. as a general massage routine.

Please be aware that these reflexes are quite tender to the touch. They should be massaged with a certain amount of pressure and stimulation in order to produce an effect. This is not subtle bodywork!

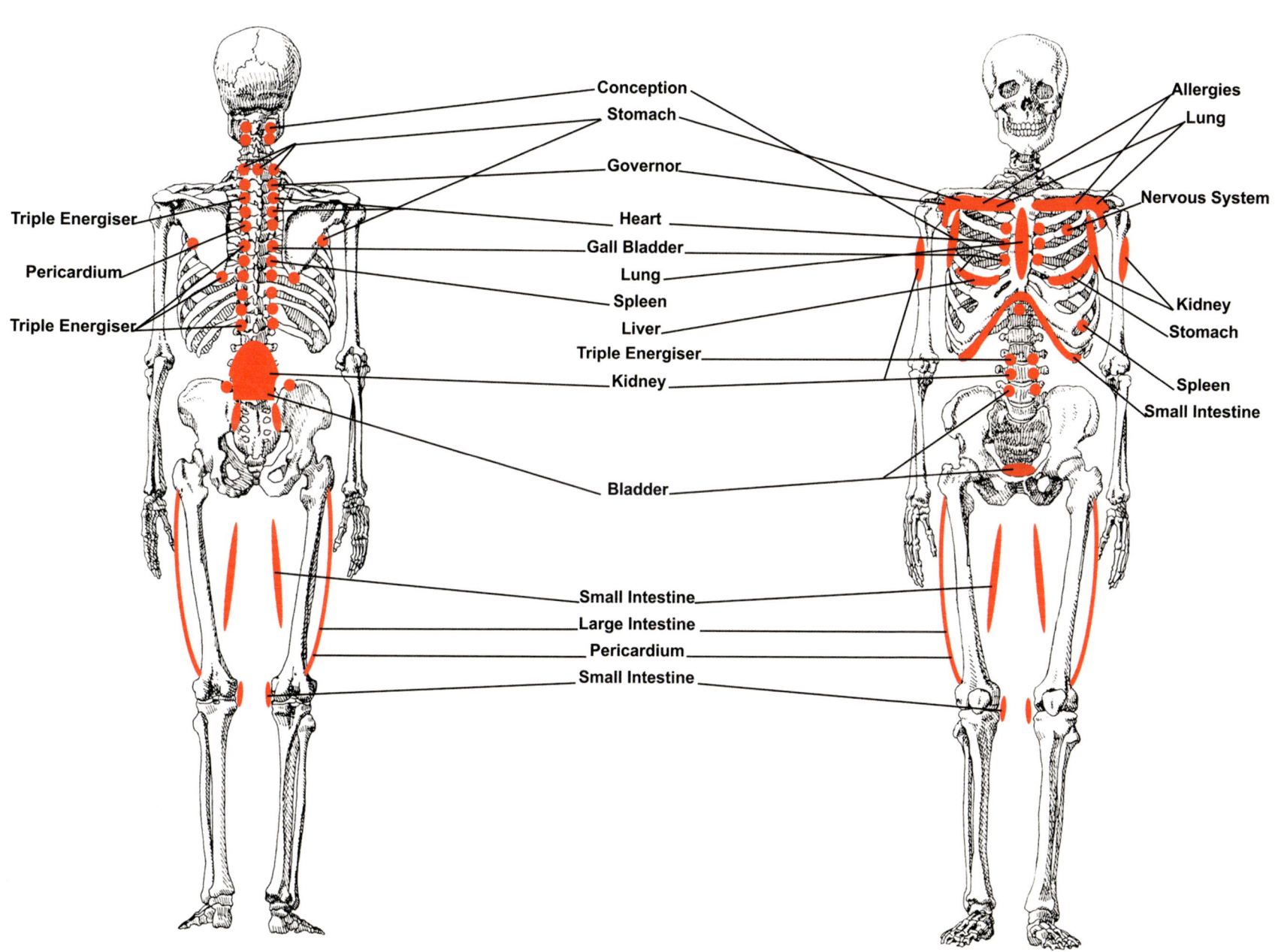

Reflected Major and Minor Chakras on the Feet and Hands

The chakras are considered to be Force Centres or whorls of energy situated from a point on the physical body and permeating through the 'layers' of the Etheric, Emotional and Mental subtle bodies of the aura in an ever increasing outward fan shaped formation. They are rotating vortices of subtle matter and are considered to be the focal points for the transmission and reception of energies. The word 'chakra' means 'wheel' in Sanskrit. To the clairvoyant, these energies may be easily seen. Each is different in form, colour and energy vibration. There are considered to be 7 major chakras and 21 minor chakras. The minor chakras are said to be reflected pathways of the majors and are closely linked to them.

The 7 major chakras have both anterior and posterior aspects along the midline of the body and are as follows:

Crown chakra	situated at the top of the head
Brow chakra	situated between the eyes
Throat chakra	situated by the throat
Heart chakra	situated in the middle of the sternum
Solar Plexus chakra	situated at the stomach
Sacral chakra	situated 2 finger-widths under the umbilicus
Base chakra	situated at the perineum

The 21 minor chakras are the Spleen, Hand, Foot, Elbow, Knee, Ear, Intercostal, Clavicular, Navel, Groin and Shoulder. The Spleen is unilateral and the remainder are bilateral.

The reflected chakras may be easily found on both the hands and feet, and their positioning mirrors their placement on the body. There are several ways of utilising the reflected chakras and they may be used in the treatment of both acute and chronic conditions.

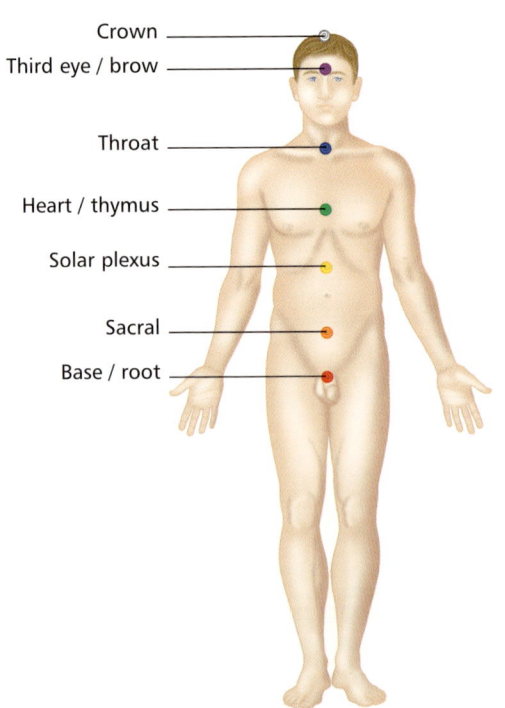

46 *Reflected Energy Pathways: A Practical Workbook for Physical Therapists*

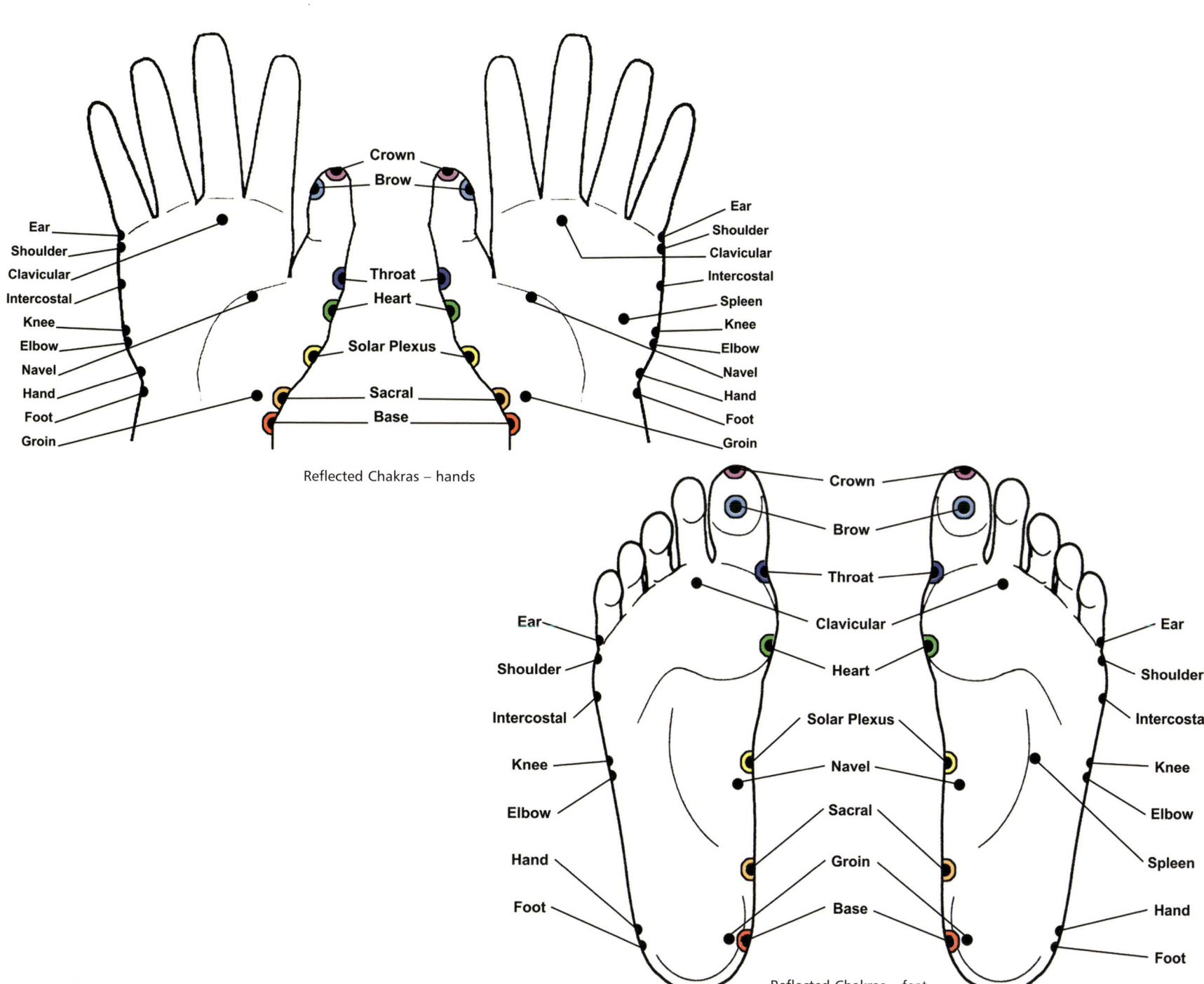

Reflected Chakras – hands

Reflected Chakras – feet

Law of Five Elements
Energy Balancing

The Law of Five Elements is one that is well known to traditional therapists the world over. It is sometimes called the Law of Five Transformations. Each of the organs/meridians is placed in one of the five 'elements' of Fire, Earth, Metal, Water and Wood – each having coupled Yin and Yang organs within each Element. I have attempted to simplify this Law in my books although in reality it is very complicated and much study is required to master all its ramifications. A simplified version of the Law is illustrated with the various associations of the individual elements.

In reflexology or acupressure it is possible to use the so-called Tonification points of each Yin and Yang meridian in order to 'energy balance' around the Sheng cycle of the circle. The opposite page shows the Tonification points on both the Yin cycle (for use in chronic conditions) and the Yang cycle (for use in acute conditions). Each remains a very useful conclusion to a treatment session. In order to energy balance, the middle finger pads are placed on any two adjacent Tonification points, e.g. LI 11 and BL 67 and held for approximately twenty seconds. Remove the hand from LI 11 and place it on the next point on the cycle – GB 43. Repeat this procedure until the whole circle is completed. An either/or situation exists in the Fire Element as there are four organ/meridians within the element.

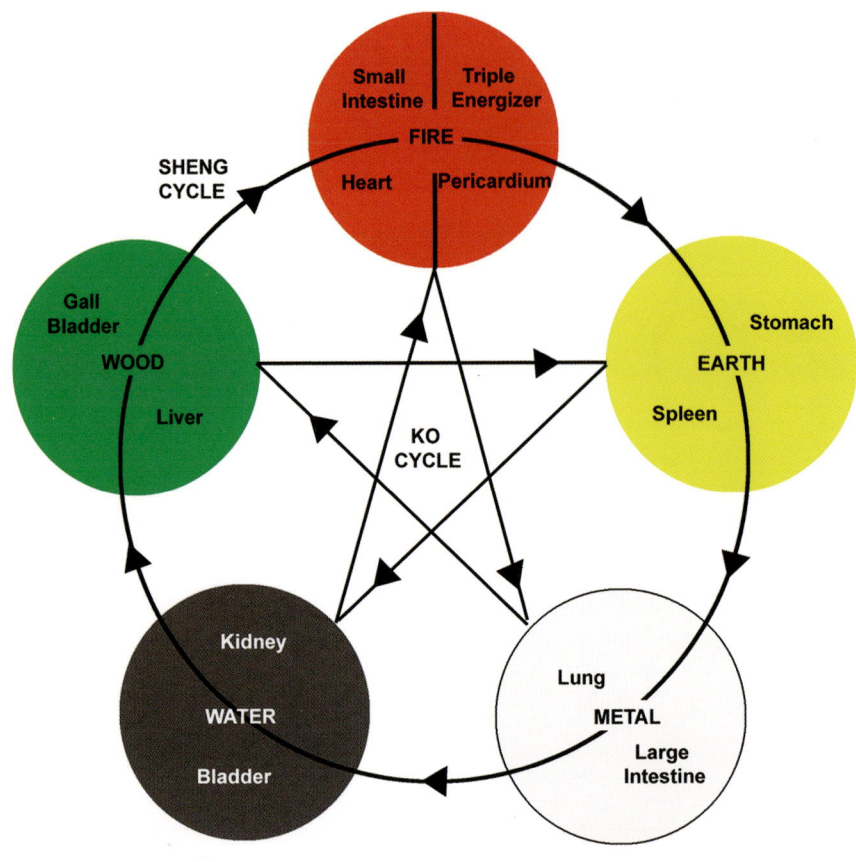

	FIRE	EARTH	METAL	WATER	WOOD
Direction	South	–	West	North	East
Colour	Red	Yellow	White	Black	Green
System	Circulation	Connective	Skin	Bone	Muscles
Face	Mouth	Tongue	Nose	Ears	Eyes
Emotion	Joy	Sympathy	Grief	Fear	Anger
Season	Summer	Late Summer	Autumn	Winter	Spring
Weather	Heat	Humidity	Dryness	Cold	Wind
Taste	Bitter	Sweet	Pungent	Putrid	Sour

48 *Reflected Energy Pathways: A Practical Workbook for Physical Therapists*

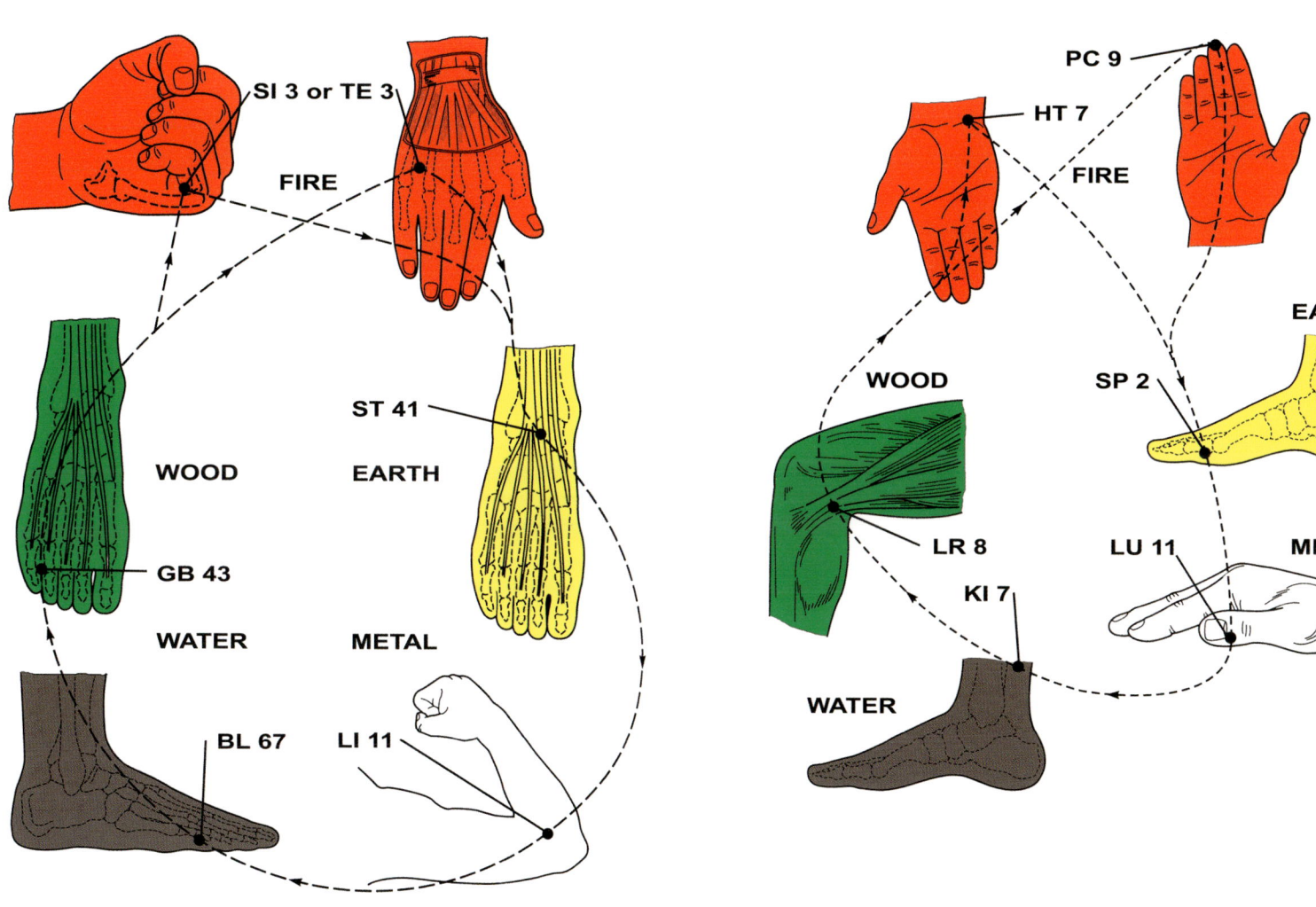

Sheng cycle energy balancing yang

Sheng cycle energy balancing yin

49

References

Charman, R.A., ed. *Complementary Therapies for Physical Therapists,* Oxford, Eng: Butterworth Heinemann, 2000

Cross, J.R. *Acupressure: Clinical Applications in Musculo-Skeletal Conditions.* Oxford, Eng: Butterworth Heinemann, 2000

Cross, J.R. *Acupressure and Reflextherapy in Medical Conditions,* Oxford, Eng: Butterworth Heinemann, 2001

Cross, J.R. *Healing with the Chakra Energy System – Acupressure, Bodywork and Reflexology for Total Health,* Berkeley, California: North Atlantic Books, 2006

Cross, J.R. *Acupuncture and the Chakra Energy System – Treating the Cause of Disease,* Berkeley, California: North Atlantic Books, July 2008

Thie, J.F. *Touch For Health: A New Approach to Restoring Our Natural Energies,* Santa Monica, California: De Vorss, 1979

Walther, D.S. *Applied Kinesiology: the Advanced Approach to Chiropractic,* Pueblo, Colorado: Systems DC, 1976